ADVANCE PRAISE

"Protecting the current and future health of our children is our collective societal responsibility and our schools provide a powerful platform to provide evidence-based health education to all of our children. Van Dusen provides a compelling blueprint for changing our attitude about health in schools across our nation."

—DR. RON DEPINHO, FOURTH PRESIDENT
OF MD ANDERSON CANCER CENTER
& FOUNDER OF OPA HEALTH

"A witty and thoughtful consideration of where education and health intersect and what the reality and possibilities are for schools. You will walk away from this book with a strong sense of urgency and purpose about the importance of health in schools!"

—JESSICA YODER, PROJECT AWARE SCHOOL-
BASED MENTAL HEALTH SPECIALIST,
INDIANA DEPARTMENT OF EDUCATION

WHEN ARE WE GOING TO TEACH HEALTH?

WHEN ARE WE GOING TO TEACH HEALTH?

LET'S TEACH HEALTH AS IF EACH CHILD'S
LIFE DEPENDS ON IT–BECAUSE IT DOES

DUNCAN VAN DUSEN

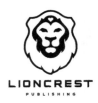

LIONCREST
PUBLISHING

WHEN ARE WE GOING TO TEACH HEALTH?
Let's Teach Health as If Each Child's Life
Depends on It – Because It Does

ISBN   978-1-5445-1713-1 *Hardcover*
      978-1-5445-0761-3 *Paperback*
      978-1-5445-0762-0 *Ebook*

To Mom & Dad

For always having your hearts in the right place and showing the courage to put your words and actions in the right place too. You are the best role models of all.

CONTENTS

Dear Reader,

I hope that you will find something obvious in this book and ask someone why it isn't being done. I also hope that you will find something nonobvious and undertake to do it.

PART I

WHY?

BENEFITS OF TEACHING HEALTH IN SCHOOLS

CHAPTER 1

———

WHAT THIS BOOK IS (AND WHAT IT ISN'T)

What follows in these pages is a synthesis of information about *why* teaching health is important to schools and children, *what* techniques make it effective, and *how* schools should integrate it as part of their core mission. This book lives at the intersection of two of our society's most pressing concerns: health and education, specifically public health and public education.

The Message and Why You Should Care

This book explains why teaching and supporting positive health behaviors should be a first-order goal of K–12 education rather than an afterthought. The case rests on two key facts which I will discuss in Part I.

First, healthy children are more productive learners, so an educational system that doesn't prioritize health education is ignoring one of the keys to its own success.

Second, the foundational behaviors of physical activity, proper nutrition, and tobacco avoidance are the key protective factors against almost all major noncommunicable diseases including diabetes, heart disease, cancer, and (with regard to the first two behaviors) obesity and Alzheimer's disease. These behaviors are also crucial to maintaining mental health and immune health, the second of which suddenly emerged as a national concern during the COVID-19 communicable disease crisis and affects whether students can even attend school. The economic and social impacts of these diseases are gargantuan and can be substantially reduced by learning basic health behaviors early in life.

Because of this disease burden, the U.S. spends more per capita on healthcare than any other country, while lagging behind other World Bank "high-income" countries in helping its citizens live long and healthy lives—measured by the World Health Organization as Healthy Life Expectancy (HALE). In 2016, the United States' HALE was 68.5 years at birth, tied for 42nd with Poland and the lowest among the 30 most economically developed countries.[1,2] In a world with overall steady increases in life expectancy, between 2010 and 2016, the United States was one of only four countries whose HALE declined. (The other three were Iraq, Libya, and Syria, all of which endured deadly civil wars during that period.) This dismal picture looks even worse when you take into account the vast life-expectancy differences and directional trends between higher- and lower-income communities in America. That gap is perhaps the exact reason our HALE falls between those of high-income and low-income countries.

We are spending too much, too late on reactive treatment of preventable disease, and it is not working well. It is time to move upstream and help a wider population avoid disease by practicing healthy habits earlier and more often. And what institution is better positioned to reach a broad swath of America's children—especially low-income ones—than our public schools? Schools are the best, and possibly only, means to ensure that all children obtain the health knowledge and skills they need for long and productive lives.

Who Should Read It?

This book is for all K–12 educators, professional or not, who collectively contribute to deciding what schools teach: principals, classroom teachers, parents of school-age children, curriculum directors, superintendents, local school boards, state and federal education policy makers and departments, and community advocates. In the U.S. alone, there are some 50 million of us, and about the same number of K–12 students. As such, one in three Americans is either a K–12 educator or a K–12 student.

What Effective Health Education Is and How Schools Can Make It Work

When schools teach health at all, they typically teach it as a supplemental class, like art, instead of as a core subject, like math. To be effective, health education needs to be given higher priority and—unlike any other subject—the way it is taught must go beyond information transfer. Effective health education *changes behavior* by shaping positive attitudes and beliefs about health, developing the social and emotional skills necessary to practice good health habits, and creating and sustaining a community that supports healthy behaviors. Health education is often called, and should really be thought of as, health promotion.

After discussing theoretical aspects of teaching health, this book describes how schools can do it more and better using the resources they already have. Schools' focus on the three foundational health behaviors of physical activity, proper nutrition, and tobacco avoidance is critical not only because they underlie so many dimensions of well-being, but also because these three health topics are the least controversial politically, and thus the best place to start.

What This Book Isn't

What follows is not a textbook on health education, because most educators don't actually read textbooks—only students and some classroom teachers do. And I guess parents sometimes do too, but only the particularly confusing parts that we are asked to explain.

Although the social, emotional, and environmental principles I discuss apply to almost every health topic,

I have chosen not to cover the entire catalog, skipping sex education, nontobacco substance abuse (i.e., alcohol, illicit, and prescription drugs), violence and injury prevention, and mental health (other than social and emotional learning). Some of these topics, in particular sex education, are highly controversial, and there are strong differences of opinion about not only what should be taught but also whether it is the schools' or parents' job to teach it.

I also don't touch a number of subjects that commonly get lumped in with school health education, such as student health services, mental health counseling, health screenings, and school staff wellness. The first three involve one-on-one healthcare, not one-to-many health education, and the last involves employee education, not student education. Although important in their own right, these topics have little to do with my central argument that health education must be integrated into the core K–12 curriculum. Muddling together everything that contains the word "health" and happens in schools distracts from a clear examination of health education and is thus an obstacle to progress.

The Messenger

I am the son of a K–12 teacher and a public health professional, and a serial entrepreneur with success in business. My current work combines all of these worlds as the founder and hands-on leader of CATCH Global Foundation, which trains schools to teach health effectively. CATCH (an acronym for Coordinated Approach To Child Health) delivers evidence-based "Whole Child" health programs, including the CATCH My Breath Youth Vaping Prevention Program, which reach approximately 15,000 schools and 3 million children around the world annually. (For more on CATCH, see chapter 10.) Over the past six years, I have consulted personally with hundreds of schools, mostly low-income Title 1 schools, on how to create a culture of health and wellness. I also speak publicly on the youth vaping epidemic and other health-related topics. My 2011 peer-reviewed research article in the *Journal of School Health* (see chapter 3) was identified by Web of Science as being in the top 1 percent of impact based on its citation count, the frequency with which other researchers reference it. And to top it off, I am the father of two teenage girls, and so my daily life is filled with conversations about what are euphemistically called "health risk behaviors."

Why Now?

Education and health have risen as both expenditures and priorities for many American families, with no end in sight. Yet the potential synergy between these two sectors, and their fundamental interdependence, have long been ignored. Just in the 12 months preceding this book's fall 2020 publication, raging epidemics of youth vaping and COVID-19 have sounded an alarm, waking many educators and parents from a long slumber on the topic of teaching health, and bringing it into the headlines and national debate. These twin crises offer all of the proof we should need that health requires education, and education requires health.

Summary

Written for K–12 educators, including parents and other decision makers, this book explains what the elements of effective health education are, why schools should provide it, and how it can fit within schools' real-life time and money constraints. I advocate for teaching health to become part of schools' core mission, for their own good and for the good of their students—both as learners now and productive adults later.

CHAPTER 2

———

PUBLIC EDUCATION AND PUBLIC HEALTH

Why these two sectors are natural partners.

Public Education in the U.S.

The first public schools opened in colonial times and are thus older than the nation itself. Our national system of public education developed in fits and starts during the 18th and 19th centuries, but by 1918 schooling was available and compulsory for all children.

Although the traditional and obvious purpose of schools is academic instruction, the National School Boards Association's description of the purpose of public education also includes "enabling students to become well-rounded individuals, focusing on the whole child and not just mastery of academic content" and "preparing students to live a productive life."

Today the primary and secondary public school system

in the United States (including charter schools), educates approximately 50 million individuals, or 90 percent of America's children in kindergarten through twelfth grade.[1] (It also educates an increasing number of pre- and even pre-pre-kindergarteners, but I'll use the traditional abbreviation K–12.) The basic structure of the system, including funding and curricular and administrative decision-making, is shown in Figure 1.

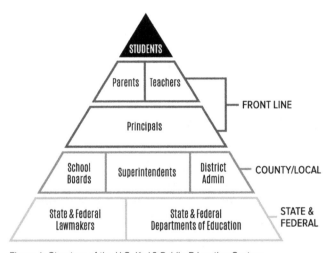

Figure 1: Structure of the U.S. K–12 Public Education System

Variations exist, sometimes including a county department of education or "intermediate district" between the state department of education and local district levels. The structure of other types of K–12 schools (including parochial, independent, and private) is generally more locally autonomous, with less regional, state, and national infrastructure.

What the Heck Is Public Health?

When my father told people he worked in public health, they nodded vaguely. As a kid, I didn't know what that meant either, so I generally avoided the subject of "what does your dad do?" with other kids. What I did know is that back in the 1970s, my dad would sometimes approach smokers and, in his Philadelphia accent, incant, "Please don't smoke. It's very bad for your health." The response to this comment was usually less vague and, from a child's perspective, utterly mortifying. So, I got my first taste of ineffective health education at an early age. If I had thought that *that* was public health, I might have avoided the subject forever.

Fortunately, as this book details, public health communications have come a long way since my dad's awkward public-service announcements and Nancy Reagan's infamous "Just Say No" antidrug campaign.

The American Public Health Association says that public health "saves money, improves our quality of life, helps children thrive, and reduces human suffering." Yet the definition of public health remains so unclear to its target audience of the general public that even graduate public health classes often start out with the question, "What is public health?" Do graduate programs in English ask students, "What is English?" I sure hope not.

In nine words, public health is wellness promotion, disease and injury prevention, and epidemiological surveillance. (And if you're wondering: epidemiological surveillance is "the ongoing, systematic collection, analysis, and interpretation of health-related data essential to planning, implementation, and evaluation of public health practice," according to the CDC.)

Public health is the fluoridated water that streams from the tap. It's the eighth and final email demanding your son's immunization record before he can enroll in school. It's the billboard warning drivers that they can't afford a DUI. It's COVID testing.

Even in normal times, you can't read the news without bumping into public health, usually on the front page or first screen. Between the opioid crisis, school shootings, changing cancer screening recommendations, and dietary scare stories, you've probably been thinking and hearing about public health a lot more and for a lot longer than you realize.

And of course, when the COVID-19 pandemic hit in early 2020, public health became all-consuming. Because the background level of public health awareness was so low, the media and governmental officials at all levels had to undertake extensive, basic educational efforts both to stanch the spread of the disease and explain what was happening. Unfortunately, in some cases this education came tinged with a dose of political partisanship, making matters much more confusing. As part of CATCH Global Foundation's "CATCH Health @ Home," in March 2020 we published a video handwashing lesson which quickly became one of our most popular resources. Wouldn't we all be better off if such basic concepts were taught proactively and systematically by professional health educators to every child in every school instead of long distance by the media, politically appointed officials, or nonprofits as a reactionary measure once a crisis is already afoot?

Encouragingly, an increasing number of young adults are learning about public health in college—the number of students graduating with a public health major grew from 1,430 in 2003 to 10,960 in 2015, a seven-and-a-half-fold rise.[2] The University of Texas at Austin, one of the largest campuses in the country, started its public health program in 2010 and as of 2020 has over 550 under-graduate majors enrolled in it.[3] Related fields, such as exercise science and nutrition, have also been among the fastest-growing majors around the country.[4] Public health is increasingly cited as a 21st-century workforce skill. In the wake of COVID-19, these trends will likely gain further momentum.

Birds of a Feather?

When you think about public education and public health together and read their statements of purpose that share concern for children and the quality and productivity of lives, you might think they operate in tandem. Unfortunately, they often don't. As we'll broach in the next chapter, recent research and thinking may provide the basis to change that for the better.

Summary

Public education and public health are both population-level efforts designed to provide components of the knowledge, skills, and safety that all citizens need for productive lives. Better coordination between these two areas of our national infrastructure is vital to the welfare of society.

CASE STUDY

Lawmakers in Action—New York City Department of Education

The school district with by far the most low-income kids in the country is in the midst of investing more than $100 million in teaching health.

New York City is the largest metropolitan area in the U.S., so it comes as little surprise that it has the nation's largest public-school system—more than 1,800 schools educating 1.1 million students.

What might be less obvious to those imagining Manhattan's glittering skyscrapers is that 73 percent of those youth are economically disadvantaged, as measured by their eligibility for federal free or reduced-price lunch (FRL) assistance, a staggering concentration of poverty.[1] New York City public schools educate more low-income students than Atlanta, Baltimore, Chicago, Cleveland, Detroit, Memphis, New Orleans, Oakland, and Philadelphia *combined*.[2]

New York City's demographics lead to many educational challenges. Recent immigrant students and their parents face language barriers; parents working multiple low-wage jobs don't have sufficient time at home to reinforce their kids' learning; families often lack reliable transportation; and they suffer the general strain of difficult economic conditions. So it is understandable that for a long time, New York City schools did not fully implement unfunded state rules around physical education and other forms of health education. But there has been a striking change in the past few years.

In 2016, Mayor Bill De Blasio's executive budget committed $100 million over four years to PE Works, whose goal is "revitalizing physical education for every student in New York City public schools and establishing physical education as a foundational component of every student's academic experience."[3,4] Overseen by the New York City Department of Education Office of School Wellness Programs, PE Works targeted all 1,600 of NYC's public schools (though not its approximately two hundred charter schools) in implementing three initiatives: investing in PE teachers, building school PE environments, and building community involvement in PE programs.

By the end of the 2018–2019 school year, PE Works had enabled the hiring and retention of 454 new licensed physical educators, giving all elementary (if not middle and high) schools at least one certified PE teacher. In addition, hundreds of preexisting PE teachers received professional development in physical education and, in turn, trained more than 12,500 classroom teachers in leading physical activity in the classroom. As discussed in chapter 8, certification and training work together to enhance teachers' ability to deliver aerobically effective physical education.

A second initiative provided 1,500 schools multiyear plans to improve PE, including specific action steps and technical assistance. In addition, 170 schools underwent facility upgrades to make PE classes safer, and the first PE lesson plan sequence for all grades was published for use throughout the district.

Finally, PE Works funded "CHAMPS" physical activity programs held before or after school and on weekends at 470 schools. The program reached more than 40,000 students; in addition, another 30,000 students participated in other supplemental programming, such as active recess, field trips, and clinics. Through these investments in staffing, training, curriculum, and environment, PE Works increased the share of students receiving the required amount of PE instruction citywide from 53 percent before the program began to 85 percent—some 350,000 more children. Data from an initial evaluation suggest the effort has led to strong and sustained improvements in students' cardiorespiratory fitness.

In 2018, the schools' chancellor made a separate $24 million investment over four years in Health Ed Works, a comprehensive health-education initiative.[5] Health Ed Works provides training and an updated, skills-development-focused curriculum for in-classroom K–12 health instruction in SEL, physical activity, nutrition, vaping prevention, personal safety, sexual health, and alcohol- and drug-use prevention.[6] The initiative also provides financial and practical support for school wellness councils, whose members work to extend a culture of health throughout the school and community environment through making policy and raising awareness of the importance of teaching health. As noted in chapter 5, skill-building and environmental support are key ingredients often missing from health education but are essential for developing positive health behaviors.

Health Ed Works currently funds a select group of 250 "Focus Schools," which include all middle schools in eight high-need neighborhoods and certain elementary, high, and special-education schools. These Focus Schools receive staff training and certification in health education, unusual since other schools in New York City (indeed, throughout the country) rarely offer health classes taught by a trained health educator. Health Ed Works also develops new standards-based curricula and supports principals and other school leaders in assigning appropriate teachers to health and in allocating sufficient time on the schedule for it. Moreover, this initiative ensures that health is taught earlier in the educational sequence than it formerly was. (As discussed in chapter 6, the timing of health education in U.S. schools is often too late to maximize its impact on long-term health behavior.) After receiving intensive assistance in implementing Health Ed Works over four years, the Focus Schools will then serve as models for the rest of the city.

Our nation's largest school district, with the most low-income kids in the country, has decided to invest approximately $25 per child per year to prioritize teaching health—because, as the next chapter will show, better health translates to better education.

CHAPTER 3

———

HEALTHY KIDS
LEARN BETTER

*Linking health education to academic
success and the Whole Child vision.*

Why Health Needs Schools

It is settled doctrine among public health professionals that schools are a crucial forum for promoting child
health. The nation's public health authority, the Centers for Disease Control and Prevention (CDC), has an
entire Division of Adolescent and School Health. Many
county health departments and community-based organizations offer programs in schools including physical
activity, nutrition and cooking, substance abuse prevention, bullying prevention, and much more.

And it's not hard to understand why. Schools are where
you can reach the most kids at once; schools are where
kids spend the majority of their waking hours; schools
are where kids get most or all of their physical activity;

and in many communities, schools are where kids get most or all of their nutrition.

Those are all reasons why health needs schools, not why schools need health. Health programs' value proposition to schools too often revolves around why we need you, not why you need us—clearly no way to get anywhere. In order to increase the priority schools place on teaching health, we need to understand and communicate the more complex reasons why teaching health can help schools.

Foundational Health Behaviors and Their Benefits

As the burden of communicable diseases like tuberculosis, smallpox, and polio has been replaced over the past century with increases in noncommunicable diseases like heart disease, cancer, obesity, diabetes, and Alzheimer's, much effort has been made to identify ways of avoiding and managing the impacts of these conditions. And in case you haven't heard, the summary advice is: exercise regularly, eat a healthy diet, and avoid tobacco.[1,2] I call these three "foundational health behaviors" and they are my priority recommendations for teaching health in K–12 schools.

Much has already been written and said about the long-term "outcome benefits" of practicing these behaviors and the fact that the earlier they are learned, the better.[3,4] Here I will focus on the set of short-term outcome and process benefits these health behaviors confer which affect education.

Practicing physical activity and healthy nutrition offers the following short-term health benefits of interest to educators.[5,6,7,8,9] Using tobacco generally has the opposite effects, so avoiding it provides these benefits too.[10,11,12,13] Numbers three and four in particular improve immune health, and numbers five through eight promote mental health.

Foundational health behaviors:

1. increase energy
2. improve blood flow, including to the brain
3. reduce microvascular inflammation
4. provide vital micronutrients including antioxidants and phytochemicals
5. reduce stress, anxiety, and depression
6. improve sleep
7. improve mood control
8. develop executive function

Why Schools Need Health

Now, of course, educators aren't officially in the business of improving blood flow or reducing stress (and students may argue the contrary on the latter). But since the late 2000s, evidence has amassed connecting foundational health behaviors directly to educational outcomes, which *are* their business.

In 2011, my graduate school research committee and I published the results of our comparison of statewide fitness and academic tests of 250,000 Texas schoolchildren in grades three through eleven.[14] The study divided kids into five groups according to their score on each of several FITNESSGRAM® tests including aerobic capacity, body-mass index (BMI), and core strength, and then looked at the comparative performance of each fitness group on the state's standardized reading and math tests, the Texas Assessment of Knowledge and Skills (TAKS). For cardiovascular fitness (a direct result of physical activity, of course), we found a significant "dose-response" correlation: each additional unit of fitness was associated with progressively higher average scores for that group on the academic tests (see figure 2). We also found no correlation between BMI and academic performance; in other words, aerobic capacity is important to educational outcomes, but body composition is not.

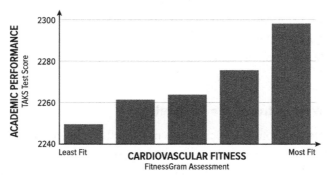

Figure 2: Correlation Between Cardiovascular Fitness and Academic Performance[15]

In 2014, the CDC analyzed the scientific research linking children's nutritious eating and adequate physical activity to academic achievement. Citing more than 60 peer-reviewed publications on the subject, the CDC identified three categories of educational benefit connected to these two crucial health behaviors:

1. better academic performance in terms of grades, standardized test scores, and graduation rates
2. better education behaviors such as attendance, discipline, and staying in school
3. better cognitive skills such as memory, concentration, and attitude[16]

Little explanation is needed as to why educators would value these results, so I'll just add that some states link school funding to attendance, giving that metric the twin benefit of better learning for students and higher revenue for the school.

The physiological benefits of diet, exercise, and tobacco avoidance clearly match up with better educational results. Increased energy and blood flow help the brain to think and remember. Better immune health improves attention and attendance. And better sleep, mood control, and executive function assist in managing behavior and concentration.

This science connects with other findings that learning is impeded when students' basic physical and emotional needs, such as food and security, are *not* being met, or if students are subject to high levels of stress or trauma from Adverse Childhood Experiences (ACEs).[17] This concept matches the famous "Hierarchy of Needs" theory developed by psychologist Abraham Maslow, which states that everyone needs to survive before they can thrive.

Schools are increasingly realizing that to perform their work, they *do* need to think about stress relief, brain function, and other dimensions of student health—but the role physical activity, nutrition, and tobacco avoidance can play in delivering them is still underappreciated.

Covering the Downside

A major concern for schools is that the academic benefits of teaching health may still not compensate for the time lost to traditional subjects. But an international review of more than one hundred published papers on the relationship between physical activity and academic achievement concluded that:

> Given competent providers, [physical activity] can be added to the school curriculum by taking time from other subjects without risk of hindering student academic achievement. On the other hand, adding time to "academic" or "curricular" subjects by taking time from physical education programmes does not enhance grades in these subjects and may be detrimental to health.[18]

In other words, using some school time at least the physical activity dimension of teaching health does not negatively affect learning outcomes in other subjects, and can actually improve academic results. (Or as I sometimes try to remind myself when I think I don't have enough time to work out, exercise makes you more productive, so it can be considered time neutral!)

A New Thought Model

So, with all of that ammunition in hand, why don't health advocates stop talking to schools about how health knowledge and practice improve health, and get to the point that health knowledge and practice improve education?

Ironically, educators seem to know this instinctively, but many only mention it once a year during standardized testing week. Have you ever heard or spoken the mantra "Get plenty of exercise and sleep the day before the test, drink water, and eat a healthy breakfast with protein and no sugar"? If that's an accepted recipe for academic performance, why aren't we using it all year round?

From "No Child Left Behind" to "Whole Child"

One reason for the discrepancy between understanding the impact of teaching health on educational success and actually implementing it is that during the same period the public health community was documenting this impact, schools were overwhelmed with trying to fulfill the requirements of the 2001 Federal "No Child Left Behind" (NCLB) legislation and countless unfunded mandates from all levels of government. Among other requirements, NCLB made schools administer annual standardized tests in reading and math to all students in third through eighth grades. Failure to meet proficiency expectations had harsh consequences for both students—who might fail to advance to the next grade level—and schools, that could be required to provide extra services such as tutoring, lose funding, or even be shut down. In that context, any subject that was not tested (like health) was often de-emphasized or cut from the school schedule.

But policy can only outrun reality for so long, and health's role in the larger educational picture continues to assert itself. The Association for Supervision and Curriculum Development (ASCD), one of the largest K–12 education associations with 113,000 superintendents, principals, teachers, and other educators in more than 125 countries, promotes a "Whole Child" model of education.[19] This philosophy seeks to change the definition of a successful student from one who is measured solely by academic test scores to one who is "emotionally and physically healthy...and ready for the world beyond formal schooling."

The Whole Child approach has five tenets: that each student be healthy, safe, engaged, supported, and challenged. These principles are also at the core of the "Whole School, Whole Community, Whole Child" (WSCC) model jointly developed by ASCD and the CDC, aligning health and education for the benefit of the child.

The term "Whole Child" is more commonly used in the world of public education; "WSCC" is more common in public health. They are essentially the same, but I favor "Whole Child" for two reasons. First, educators are the decision makers about what gets taught in schools, so it's better to use a term that already has currency with them. Second, "Whole Child" to some degree defines itself, whereas "WSCC" requires explanation to many educators, to say nothing of the general public. Anyway, who needs another acronym when plain English will do?

Though it's difficult to quantify the breadth of reforms it has inspired, it is safe to say that the Whole Child concept has affected and entered into the vocabulary of thousands of schools. Of the 10 largest districts in the country, which collectively educate almost 10 percent of the nation's schoolchildren, five specifically include "Whole Child" in their mission statements, core values, or other high-level goals, and three others use the term in more narrow contexts. As mentioned in chapter 1, the National School Boards Association also uses "Whole Child" in its description of the very purpose of public education. Although much work remains on the "what" and "how" of teaching health, the adoption of Whole Child principles in schools constitutes progress in agreeing on the "why."

Whole Child thus represents a common cause between educators and public health professionals—a shared paradigm embracing the vision that health education not only improves health; it improves education.

Summary

Schools should teach health because it provides immediate benefits that drive learning behaviors and academic success, not to mention the longer-term economic and quality-of-life benefits of disease avoidance. The Whole Child model, which many schools and districts have incorporated into their strategic thinking, provides a conceptual basis for prioritizing health.

Recommended Actions

Parents of school-age children: Band together to advocate for health education to your school principal. Cite the connections between health and learning and the term "Whole Child," especially if it is part of your district or school's mission or strategic plan.

Teachers: Teach health with the passion, personal commitment, and student accountability that you put into other subjects.

Principals: Understand and consider the mounting evidence that health impacts academic success.

School boards, superintendents, and district administrators: Require the teaching of health in all K–12 schools, especially physical education, nutrition education, and especially in elementary schools.

Lawmakers and education policy makers: Devise policies and incentives that drive schools to actively own, not just allow, health education.

CASE STUDY

Principal in Action—Solomon P. Ortiz Elementary School, Brownsville, Texas

A Texas principal credits her school's top academic standing to a focus on teaching health.

Ortiz Elementary sits at the southernmost tip of Texas in Brownsville, just six thousand feet from the Rio Grande and the U.S. border with Mexico. Its students are virtually all low income (92 percent) as measured by their eligibility for federal free or reduced-price lunch (FRL) assistance. As is unfortunately typical of such low-income areas, the community bears a high burden of obesity and diabetes.[1]

The region around Brownsville has grown rapidly since the passage of NAFTA in 1994, becoming a major automotive manufacturing and transportation hub. Like many Texas border towns, Brownsville is dwarfed by a neighbor city across the bridge in Mexico, Matamoros, with triple its population. The combined metropolitan areas of these two cities include approximately 1.5 million people—about the size of Jacksonville or Milwaukee.

Brownsville's population is overwhelmingly Hispanic and follows many Latino food, holiday, social, and cultural traditions. According to the 2010 Census, Brownsville's per-capita income of $10,960 was the third lowest of the 276 largest cities in the United States— but it was ranked as the safest of 24 Texas cities included in the FBI's 2013 Uniform Crime Reports.[2]

Ortiz might be expected to be a low-performing school based on the disconcerting correlation between lower incomes and lower academic performance in Texas public schools. This association is clearly visible when FRL eligibility is compared with the Texas Education Agency (TEA) Accountability Rating system, which grades three measures of academic success from "A" to "F" (see figure 3, using a standard 4.0 GPA scale).[3]

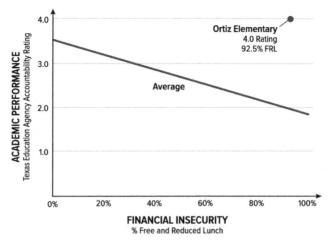

Figure 3: Correlation between Economic Status and School Ratings among Texas Public Schools

Beating the Educational Odds

Yet Ortiz has managed to beat these long educational odds. It was:

- among only 6 percent of Texas public schools that earned the equivalent of a 4.0 GPA in the 2018–2019 TEA Accountability Rating,[4] which considers a variety of indicators, such as graduation rates, college, career, and military readiness, SAT/ACT scores, and college prep course completion
- among only 30 schools statewide (0.05 percent of Texas public schools) with 92 percent or higher FRL eligibility that earned a 4.0 Accountability Rating that year
- 1 of 11 schools recognized by the TEA as a High Performing and High Progress Title 1 School in 2014–2015[5]

- 1 of 15 schools nationally to win the National Center for Urban School Transformation's America's Best Urban Schools Award in both 2015 and 2018[6]

How did they do it?

Personal and Community Involvement in Promoting a Culture of Health

To hear Principal Patricia Garza answer this question is to listen to a passionate testimonial on the educational and redemptive power of a culture of health. "Ortiz looks at the whole child, not just their brains," she says. "When kids can also use their bodies to excel, that gives them confidence in the classroom, transforming them through higher self-esteem and respect from peers and teachers."

Before serving as principal, Garza was Ortiz's dean of instruction and pushed hard to increase the schools' academic rigor. She developed clearer and more demanding expectations of students in the primary grades, especially in reading and writing. She also observed closely what holds kids back, which led her to guide Ortiz in integrating special-needs kids into classes with their peers and increasing opportunities for all kids to participate in physical activity and other health behaviors.

Garza's entire staff of teachers, administrators, and other professionals reports to school at 7:30 a.m. each weekday so they can supervise a variety of before-school activities. The most popular is a running and fitness club with an average daily attendance of 230 kids—almost half the student body! Garza set the club in motion by enlisting an enthusiastic teacher, whose positivity was contagious among students. As the club grew, the school occasionally had to cap participation to sustain a safe staff-to-student ratio. Responding to the demand, parents and other community members quickly signed on as volunteers, and Garza redeployed paraprofessionals to help out as well. This all-hands approach ensured that the club could stay open to all without adding a penny to the school's budget.

Among the club's many benefits is that vigorous activity before school helps kids get settled for a day of learning. In particular, the club has enabled a large population of students diagnosed with ADHD to manage their condition with minimal or no medication. Garza has observed that kids who previously couldn't stay in their seats have greatly improved their concentration and, as a result, their grades.

She also ensured that Ortiz Elementary takes full advantage of the lunchroom as a health-education classroom. Students in kindergarten through second grade enjoy special cafeteria tours, and all students are served nutritious snacks that rotate with the seasons. Along the way, they learn about the negative effects of food processing and added sugar and salt, among other topics. In the cafeteria and elsewhere, the school environment surrounds students with health information, including posters featuring the simple and memorable GO-SLOW-WHOA food classification system (see chapter 9).

So important is the lunchroom to the school culture that Principal Garza takes a cafeteria shift every day. She greets cafeteria workers, thanking them for their efforts to keep kids healthy, and talks to students about what they're eating, why it is (or isn't) a healthy choice, and what their favorite fruits and vegetables are. She also seats herself where everyone can watch her eat her own healthy lunch—Social Cognitive Theory in action! (See chapter 5.)

At Ortiz, health is a team sport. The school has a wellness team that meets once per six-week grading period (see chapter 6) and recruits additional players from the community by engaging parents in its health programming. Garza says that many of these parents tell her they want to provide a healthier environment for their kids, but lack education in how to do so—especially on a tight budget. She has made bridging that knowledge and skill gap a key part of Ortiz's mission, regularly sending health messages home with students and organizing health-oriented parent events and programs.

For example, each year Ortiz holds a very well-attended "Family Fun Night" that offers healthy foods and physical activities parents can enjoy with their kids. The school also had the kids create and wear "heavenly hats" as tributes to people fighting cancer in a parade the school staged as a cancer-awareness event. It drew enthusiastic participation from both students and parents, and the entry fees (one dollar per hat) were donated to local cancer patients.

One important attribute all these student health initiatives have in common: they drain little, if any, extra money from the school budget. Principal Garza resourcefully deployed her own and her staff's existing time, selected activities that could be done with existing equipment, and marshalled contributions of volunteer time and materials from the community. Garza cultivated this involvement by creatively recognizing exceptional volunteers. For example, in 2018 she thanked them in a special ceremony complete with students dressed up as cheerleaders.

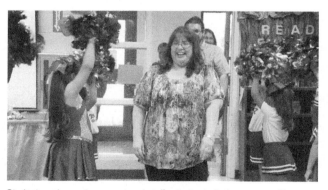

Students welcome top parent and staff volunteers during a recognition ceremony (Photograph by Brownsville ISD. Used with permission. Full video at https://youtu.be/6u17yo2ou2Y.)

A Word to the Wise

Is there really a connection between Ortiz's prioritizing Whole Child health and its students' academic success?

Garza has no doubt: "Absolutely!" Her closing advice to other principals:

> If you are analyzing how to improve your school's performance, look at the bottom kids and consider whether better health could help them. If you say you don't have time to teach health, you are not using your time efficiently, because health may, in fact, be the solution you are looking for.

CHAPTER 4

BARRIERS TO
TEACHING HEALTH

Why health education is hard to do in our K–12 schools.

With all of the good reasons for integrating health education into the K–12 curriculum, why isn't it more of a priority in our public education system? To answer that question, we need to look beyond bromides like "not enough time" and "not enough money," which are symptoms of the lack of priority, not explanations for it.

The barriers to teaching health fall into two main categories: structural and philosophical.

Structural Barriers

For better or worse, the structure of the American primary and secondary educational system is highly distributed (see chapter 2, figure 1). School funding, governance, curricular decision-making, and accountability are spread among many separate hands. What's more, their mechanisms are different in each of the several types of school: public, charter, parochial, and private (most but not all "independent" schools). Even within the largest category, public schools, the organizational unit—the school district—ranges in size from a few dozen students to more than a million, and the level of central control varies widely. Some districts operate with a top-down structure, while others give principals much more autonomy.

Such a distributed system penalizes health education by having both too many and too few chiefs. The many chiefs impose mandates on schools that others are expected to fund, and whose collective budget and time requirements exceed the bounds of physics. In this context, finding resources to fund and implement the study of subjects that aren't required, such as health, is very hard. At the same time, every actor in this system can legitimately claim they are not a chief and that they have too little power to overcome structural inertia and experiment with a new idea like stronger health education.

These dynamics can lead to infinite catch-22s, which make it difficult for anyone to initiate change. The federal government cannot require more health education, because it's up to the states and the schools to decide, but the states and the schools cannot implement more health education because the federal government will neither provide them more money nor eliminate any current requirements in return. The College Board and the state boards of education do not test health seriously, because it's not taught seriously, and schools don't teach it seriously because it's not tested seriously. In other words, it's difficult to make health education a priority because it isn't already a priority.

Philosophical Barriers

The other category of barriers to health education is philosophical. In general, it is simply not considered as important as other subjects, so it loses out in the competition for a limited pool of time and money. Why is that?

One explanation stems from an abiding, almost subconscious perception that good health practices are common sense: "Kids all know that tobacco is bad for you, so why waste valuable school minutes reiterating that fact?" Yet despite the success of many years of sophisticated tobacco-control efforts in the U.S., the youth vaping crisis has demonstrated how suddenly such a danger can reappear without consistent prevention efforts targeting youth (see chapter 7). If health behaviors are indeed common sense, why, in our increasingly wealthy and technologically sophisticated society, are life expectancy and HALE shrinking?[1] Clearly, if people were going to figure out good health on their own, they already would have.

A more subtle and perhaps more insidious excuse for not teaching health in schools is the largely unspoken sense that health behaviors are an oral and social tradition whose norms parents and community members are responsible for imparting to children. The most obvious example of this belief is sex education, but it extends to other health behaviors too. Because health is already built into public policy and communication and is thus already part of the basic infrastructure of society, the task of our schools—so the thinking goes—is to educate kids in the more esoteric topics parents aren't equipped to teach. But in reality, few parents are equipped to teach health properly either, even with the workshops and support that some schools are beginning to offer.

The fact that our society mostly leaves health education to families and communities may help explain the vexing "health disparities" that accompany entrenched economic and educational disparities throughout the country. (On the other hand, there is no reason to believe that all privileged families are successful at teaching health at home either.) These "social determinants of health"—and the fact that areas with lower economic and educational status also tend to have lower health status—are a major social justice issue. Not all kids have parents who are willing and able to teach health, but all kids have a school. If our schools cannot ensure that every child gets the health education they need, who will?

Our Prevention Blind Spot

The fact that health education is marginalized in K–12 schools reflects our society's reactive, short-term philosophy about health in general.

Every dollar spent on health prevention returns up to five dollars in disease cost avoidance and untold value in quality and length of life.[2] So the minutes of school productivity "lost" to preventive health education and behaviors are actually free, or at least much less expensive, than paying for sickness through days lost.

Yet of our $3.3 trillion annual healthcare tab in the United States, only 9 percent is spent on prevention, while 91 percent is spent on treatment.[3,4] And of these prevention dollars, less than half go toward "primary" prevention, or preventing problems from happening in the first place. The remainder is allocated to "secondary" prevention, screenings, and disease management for early detection and mitigation. Perhaps it is only natural that our schools reflect the low priority our society gives to prevention.

We believe return-on-investment (ROI) arguments for our spending on technology, on home improvement, and on taking vacations. And we clearly believe in the ROI of education in general—the whole system runs on trading years of economic productivity for larger future gains created by an educated populace. So why do we have such a hard time believing that investments in teaching health will pay off too?

All of these barriers can and must be overcome. The next two parts of this book will talk about what schools can do and how, much of which is possible within current time and budget constraints.

Summary

Health education suffers from the inertia built into the decentralized structure of our K–12 school system and a philosophical mindset that it isn't really the schools' role to teach health. Individual actors are often unwilling or unable to meaningfully prioritize teaching health.

PART II

WHAT?

THEORIES BEHIND TEACHING HEALTH EFFECTIVELY

CHAPTER 5

THE RECIPE FOR EFFECTIVE HEALTH EDUCATION

The teaching strategies needed to move beyond knowledge acquisition to health-behavior acquisition.

Two theories of human behavior are crucial to understanding what makes health teaching effective: Social Cognitive Theory (SCT) and Diffusion of Innovations Theory (DOI). This chapter provides a primer in each and serves as a crucial bridge between abstraction and practicality. These theories are indispensable to understanding which health education techniques work, and why—and we will return to them repeatedly as we delve deeper. In the recipe for effective health education, SCT guides the ingredients and DOI guides the procedure.

Health Is about Behavior

It is natural to assume that the goal of health education,

like education in traditional classroom subjects, is simply the transmission of knowledge and that students can and will transform the knowledge they acquire into healthy actions on their own. But as we're about to discuss, the relationship between knowledge and behavior change is weak. Presumably, we aren't offering health education solely as a dispassionate means of imparting facts, but out of a moral and social duty to condition youth toward healthy behaviors and away from risky ones. So, it follows that the real goal of health education is not knowledge acquisition but *behavior acquisition*—making health unique among educational subjects.

Social Cognitive Theory: A Model of Behavioral Learning

Because health education has a different goal, we also need to employ different teaching methods for it, using models proven in behavioral science research. One of the most widely accepted of these models is SCT, which is a scientific name for a principle everybody knows: Monkey see, monkey do. All of us, especially children, identify role models, and our behavior is shaped more by what they do than by what they say, or by our knowledge of abstract facts.

SCT identifies three factors that determine how people learn and then repeat a specific behavior:

- Personal: what do I know, what can I do, and what are my attitudes and beliefs about doing those things?

- Social: what is the social response I receive from other people when performing the behavior, and what do I learn from the social practice of the behavior?
- Environmental: how does my environment support and reward or punish the behavior?

SCT is often communicated using an equilateral triangle, with each of these factors at the points and behavior in the middle (see figure 4). The factors are all equally important and necessary to supporting behavior.

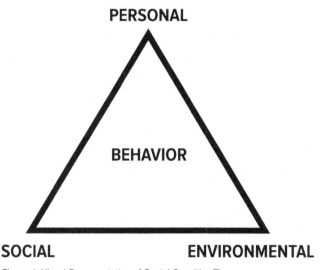

Figure 4: Visual Representation of Social Cognitive Theory

Psychologist Albert Bandura's original experiments, which led to his development of SCT, involved showing children video footage of other children hitting a "Bobo doll." Noticing that kids were more likely to display aggressive behavior after watching their peers punching Bobo, Bandura concluded that demonstration is a vital part of learning—and adopting—new behaviors. (A point you are unlikely to hear from makers of violent movies and video games.)

Implications of SCT for Health Education

Since the goal of health education is shaping behavior, the measure of its success also needs to be behavior. In other words, a person who has outstanding knowledge of health but lacks the motivation, ability, confidence, or support to engage in positive health behaviors in effect has a *low* level of health education. On the other hand, someone who has less factual knowledge but has skills, positive health beliefs, and a supportive environment can be said to have a *high* level of health education. In this sense, health education could be called "health proficiency." So, a school whose health education program focuses solely on health knowledge and ignores the other SCT components of attitude building, personal-skill building, social-skill building, and environmental support is likely to be disappointed with the health behavior that results.[1]

For example, telling children that vegetables are healthy and that they should eat more of them is far less effective in increasing their vegetable consumption than strategies such as:

- modeling vegetable consumption and enjoyment by an admired adult like a principal or parent
- discussing what they think about vegetables and why
- having them taste different vegetables
- teaching them to plant and harvest vegetables
- artfully displaying vegetables in the cafeteria
- encouraging creativity in naming vegetables and explaining their benefits on signs or posters
- providing positive reinforcement for eating vegetables.

This range of activities more fully covers the attitude development, skill-building, social feedback, and environmental support that SCT recommends for learning and sustaining positive health behaviors.

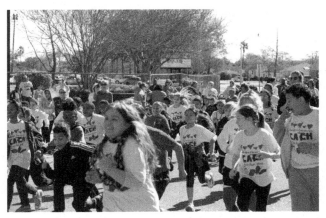

SCT in action: Kids' Fun Run at Audubon Elementary School, New Orleans with support and participation from adults. (Note homemade CATCH T-shirts; see chapter 10.) (Photograph by Jefferson Parish Schools. Used with permission.)

SCT Meets SEL

You may have already noted that SCT's inclusion of environment (which is social) and attitudes and beliefs (which are, essentially, emotions) overlaps an educational framework many schools already use: Social and Emotional Learning (SEL). The Collaborative for Academic, Social, and Emotional Learning (CASEL) has been working for more than 20 years to define SEL and ensure that it is integrated into education.[2] This model is organized around five competencies: self-awareness, self-management, social awareness, relationship skills, and responsible decision-making. We can combine these terms as follows: SCT says that health behavior is driven by the combination of health knowledge acquisition, development of SEL skills to apply that knowledge, and establishment of a socially rewarding environment.

This principle has been amply demonstrated in assessment of youth tobacco-prevention education programs. As shown in a 1999 study, knowledge of tobacco's harmful effects, by itself, has little connection to reduced experimentation and product use.[3] Classroom time is better spent on SEL and skill-building topics, such as expressing personal goals and how tobacco addiction interferes with achieving them; identifying manipulative media techniques designed to promote the myth that tobacco is glamorous and fun; and developing refusal strategies with peers that don't make kids feel like complete dorks.

These youth empowerment-oriented approaches have

demonstrated effectiveness and have gained currency in education circles under the broader terms "active learning" or the "flipped" or "inverted" classroom.[4] In these teaching models, students first digest facts on their own as homework, and then spend their class time in group problem-solving, discussion, and elaboration. This teaching style is a modern extension of the classic Socratic method of guided learning, in which teachers ask students questions rather than reciting facts. For example, in vaping prevention, instead of saying, "Vaping harms lung function," asking, "What effects could vaping have on your body?" and "How could that affect your personal goals?" It is surely no surprise to educators and parents that empowerment is a significantly more successful approach to reaching today's youth than authoritarian lecturing.

Diffusion of Innovations Theory: Spreading the Word

While SCT provides a good model for learning health behavior at an individual level, DOI helps educators plan how to propel that learning across many individuals or groups at the population level. SCT shows that learning is based on observing models; DOI shows which models we choose. The basic principle of DOI is that new ideas and devices are adopted through a process of change that proceeds systematically through specific segments of the population. Some people want to be the "first on the block" to have a new gadget. These are the "Innovators." Others want to hear how that person likes it before they get it but still beat everyone else to the store ("Early Adopters"). Still others want to see a good number of people use it and work out the kinks before they jump on the bandwagon (the "Majority"). Finally, those who still like their flip phone just fine and are waiting a few more years to see if the smartphone fad blows over are the "Laggards."

DOI is often represented by a bell curve, with Innovators on the left side and Laggards on the right—essentially a left-to-right timeline of adoption. The reason a bell curve is used is because the adoption groups are of very different sizes. Importantly, the Innovators and Early Adopters (together, "thought leaders") that are in the shaded area to the left of the vertical line in figure 5 represent only 1/6, or 17 percent, of the population.

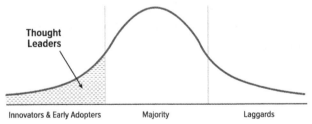

Figure 5: Visual Representation of Diffusion of Innovations Theory

According to DOI, the key to spreading any new concept is to identify that minority of thought leaders in a group, introduce them to the idea first, get them to embrace it, and then let them take the lead in evangelizing about it to everyone else. Teachers creating discussion groups in health class should empower thought-leader students to be their moderators; principals forming School Wellness Teams (see chapter 6) should pick thought-leader teachers as team leaders; districts seeking to spread the teaching of health across a school system should pilot it at thought-leader schools. Of course, the kind of thought leaders you want for these purposes are not just the ones willing to go first, but the ones who also inspire followers.

When it comes to teaching health (or anything else, for that matter), the thought leader is often not the one with the leadership title. So, how do you identify thought leaders? One simple and powerful way is to just ask members of a community, "Who are the thought leaders around here?" or a variation, such as, "Who often has an idea first?" or "Who gives you your best ideas?" You can also observe social interactions, looking for people with "informal status," i.e., those whose ideas and actions command the most attention independent of their formal rank. A third excellent test is to notice what kind of questions people ask. Thought leaders evaluate concepts for novelty and opportunity and can "suspend disbelief" on details; members of the Majority and Laggards ask about process details and want references and reviews from others who have gone before them.

Remember, according to DOI, approximately one in six members of a group are thought leaders, so if you are identifying a much higher or lower proportion, you may want to reconsider. It is also important to note that people do not fall into the same DOI stage in all aspects of life. For example, yours truly is an Innovator when it comes to ideas, an Early Adopter when it comes to books, and in the Majority (Late Majority if we're being honest) when it comes to gadgets. So don't necessarily mistake the fashion leader, the technology leader, or the music leader for the thought leader.

Recipe for Effective Health Education

What is the appropriate balance of SCT ingredients for teaching health effectively? In 1995, the first version of the National Health Education Standards (NHES) was published, providing a framework to help teachers, curriculum developers, and policy makers deliver and assess K–12 health education.[5] It has since become the accepted model and was updated in the mid-2000s. The eight NHES standards are:

1. Students will comprehend concepts related to health promotion and disease prevention to enhance health.
2. Students will analyze the influence of family, peers, culture, media, technology, and other factors on health behaviors.
3. Students will demonstrate the ability to access valid information, products, and services to enhance health.
4. Students will demonstrate the ability to use interpersonal communication skills to enhance health and avoid or reduce health risks.
5. Students will demonstrate the ability to use decision-making skills to enhance health.

6. Students will demonstrate the ability to use goal-setting skills to enhance health.
7. Students will demonstrate the ability to practice health-enhancing behaviors and avoid or reduce health risks.
8. Students will demonstrate the ability to advocate for personal, family, and community health.

Notice that only two of the standards (numbers one and three) relate primarily to digesting information. The other six involve building personal and social competencies. In other words, the NHES standards give SEL and environmental components *three times* the weight of factual knowledge in terms of the expected outcomes for health education.

As an example of applying these proportions, the evidence-based CATCH My Breath youth vaping prevention program (see chapters 7 and 10) devotes only one of four lessons to health facts and the rest to correcting misperceptions about social norms, practicing refusal skills, and reducing students' emotional susceptibility to experimentation. The program provides posters, videos, and parent education as environmental support. It also furnishes starter materials to allow youth to develop agency and reinforce learning through anti-vaping community service projects. These teen-led projects enable students to build an environment of health by delivering community presentations, creating and communicating counter-advertising, and engaging with policy-making authorities (see the case study on a "Student in Action" for an example).

The need for SEL and environmental components in school health education means that achieving effectiveness will take a lot more than finding a decent teacher and building a facts-based curriculum.[6] Unfortunately, most schools are unaware of the importance of a more holistic approach or how to deploy it. A CDC survey determined that throughout our nation's schools, the majority of health instruction provides *no* opportunity for activities outside of knowledge exchange, such as practicing "communication, decision-making, goal setting, or refusal skills."[7] Fixing this common imbalance between teaching facts and addressing the wider determinants of health behavior (SEL skills, social norms, and environment) is essential to making school health education more effective.

Research on Health Education Practices

The best and worst practices in youth substance abuse prevention were summarized in an October 2016 guide published by the State of Washington designed for health departments and school and community health educators.[8] This synthesis of research from more than 50 academic papers should humble anyone who believes that devising effective health education requires only common sense.

The report's focus is on strategies for teaching negative

behavior avoidance (e.g., not using alcohol, drugs, and other substances), but its recommendations also pertain to training youth in positive health behaviors (e.g., being physically active and choosing nutritious foods). Over the past three years, the guide has been distributed to thousands of people, and the state's Health Care Authority receives regular requests for it from around the country.

Best Practices

The most effective prevention strategies the state of Washington identifies align with SCT and SEL principles. Among the best practices for teaching health, they cite:

- building social and personal skills
- identifying immediate rather than long-term consequences of unhealthy behavior (e.g., smoking stains your teeth, rather than smoking causes cancer)
- communicating positive peer norms
- involving youth with peer-led components, and
- using interactive approaches to practice and reinforce skills.

Perhaps most interesting on this list of strategies is the deafening silence around imparting knowledge—reinforcing that when it comes to health, the importance of facts is dwarfed by having the right attitudes, beliefs, and behavioral skills to act on those facts. This principle may seem counterintuitive, but again, we wouldn't need science if everything was common sense.

Worst Practices

The guide's lead author, Monroe Community Coalition Coordinator Joe Neigel, makes the important point that the guide's list of what *not* to do includes health education practices that are not only ineffective but also counterproductive. In other words, such efforts may inadvertently encourage the unhealthy behaviors they are hoped to prevent.

"Fear-arousal," including presenting gruesome images and sensationalized dangers, tops his list of common mistakes. Teens' own real-world experiences may make this information seem exaggerated, which leads them to discredit the messenger or creates a desire to prove adults wrong. It should be noted that inciting fear in health communications does have some evidence of success. For example, research has shown that using graphic warning labels seems to deter adults from smoking.[9,10] But with a delicate balance of pros and cons, this technique is better left to health communications professionals; schools should not use fear as a cornerstone of health education but focus instead on the skill-building and environmental factors we have discussed.

Another tactic to avoid is one-time assemblies warning kids off substance use. These events are at best little-remembered and ineffective. When combined with fear arousal—for example, "mock car crashes" to teach the dangers of drunk driving—such presentations can induce trauma and increase risky behavior, working least well with the members of the audience who need help the most.

The guide goes on to describe research showing that knowledge-only interventions, including fact sheets and common "myth-busting" techniques, are the least effective ways to teach health behaviors and may even encourage defiance and experimentation. Our minds often remember myths as facts, so it's best not to state them in the first place. Moralizing appeals may also backfire, because a teenager's process of identity formation involves challenging established values such as "drugs are bad!"

Finally, and again counterintuitively, behavioral science research cited in the guide has documented the dangers of presenting youth with the personal testimony of people in recovery. Although the individual will likely describe how bad substance abuse made their life, they will also model the beneficial results of healing and the positive attention that comes from it. The person's end result of personal growth can easily overshadow their original problem of addiction, leaving listeners with the wrong message. On the other hand, hearing stories from survivors of mental health crises has been shown to help teens internalize positive examples of hope and comradeship to counter feelings of futility and isolation.

A key takeaway from this excellent resource is that schools should carefully hew to health education programs with scientific evidence of effectiveness rather than relying on material only because it is commonly used or seems like it will help.

Summary

Health is fundamentally different from other school subjects because its goal is not knowledge acquisition but behavior acquisition. SCT demonstrates that in addition to imparting information, effective health education must create a healthy environment and teach the application of social and emotional skills, such as self-awareness, self-efficacy, and socially competent refusal. Principles from DOI can accelerate the process of teaching health by empowering thought leaders to evangelize for behavior norms across a social group.

Recommended Actions

Parents of school-age children: In addition to discussing health facts, rehearse attitudes and social skills related to health with your children. Consider the health behaviors you are modeling at home.

Principals, superintendents, and district administrators: Provide regular training and professional development for teachers on how to deliver effective health education that includes skill-building and social and emotional learning. Be systematic in identifying and empowering thought leaders.

Lawmakers and education policy makers: Codify the

definition of "health education" as addressing both knowledge and behavior acquisition.

CASE STUDY

Parents in Action—GROW Central Florida

A parent grows from being a solo volunteer to starting an organization to train and mobilize other parents to support health programs in schools.

The story of Colleen Gonzalez and GROW Central Florida began modestly enough. In 2009, after a decade of experience in corporate human resources, Gonzalez left her job to become a stay-at-home mom. Seeking to become more involved in her child's Seminole County, Florida school, she started volunteering to help with health programming. By 2015, her work had evolved to coaching and organizing other parent volunteers. That year, she founded GROW Central Florida, a 501(c)(3) nonprofit whose acronym stands for Grass Roots Outreach Within. A public school parent-outreach organization, GROW works to promote environments that support increased opportunities for physical activity and healthy living for Central Florida schoolchildren by partnering with grassroots volunteers and unfunded school health and wellness programs. By 2018, running GROW had become Gonzalez's full-time job.

As of 2020, GROW boasts a $150,000 annual budget, mobilizes more than 80 volunteers at 47 schools, and reaches approximately 13,500 elementary school kids per year through several programs. The organization is proof that motivated parents can drive health education by thinking outside the usual bounds of simply asking for more dollars and minutes for it.

Action and Impact

Not impressed with "PTAs having cookie sales," Gonzalez began observing what was happening at other area schools. Some had running clubs, so she offered to start a before-school cross-country club at Lake Orienta Elementary School. The school initially declined the offer but let her arrange for student participation in National Walk-to-School Day and a monthly "Walk & Roll" program. Gonzalez's efforts proved so successful and Gonzalez so trustworthy that the next year, the school did allow her to create a student running club. The first year, 40 runners enrolled, and more than one hundred participated in its second year.

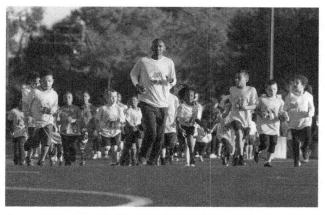

Teamwork! (Photograph by Eric Padgett. Used with permission.)

Today, supporting volunteer running coaches and unfunded teams is GROW Central Florida's signature service. As of the 2019–2020 school year, the running program has grown to include participation by all of Seminole County's 37 public elementary schools and two charter schools, reaching a total of 5,618 kids ages five to twelve who train with 74 volunteer coaches. GROW also supported volunteer race directors who held nine meets with a total of 8,500 runners. GROW volunteers help organize the schedule and awards ceremony and the GROW organization provides the logistical support for event management as well as durable goods such as loudspeakers and flags bought with donations. In a before-and-after survey the same year, 564 parents of running club members reported that as a result of participating, their children had increased their daily physical activity by an average of 21 minutes (from 58 to 79 minutes per child per day), with all children getting at least 30 minutes of exercise per day.

According to the parents, the emotional impact of GROW's program has been as significant as its physical impact. Parent Janine Morse says:

> I love this organization! My son, who has autism, participated in Runner's Club for the first time this year at school, and I was hesitant about letting him participate in the races because I thought he would get upset if he could not keep up with the other kids. I am so thankful that his PE teacher, Coach Segrest, encouraged me to let him participate in the races and reassured me that she would run with him so he would not be by himself. Landon loved participating in all the races and was so happy when he beat Coach Segrest across the finish line.

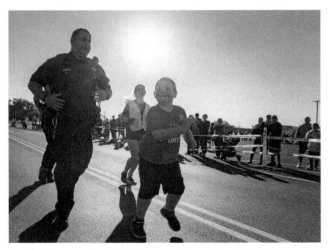

Landon Morse runs in a GROW-sponsored race with a School Resource Deputy (Photograph by GROW Central Florida. Used with permission.)

As an extension of this program, GROW began providing shoes for students in need of proper athletic footwear. A collaboration with Fleet Feet Orlando, a local shoe retailer, initially yielded donations of 20 to 30 pairs at a time. GROW Central Florida and Fleet Feet Orlando were later spotlighted at a Fleet Feet corporate meeting, which inspired footwear companies New Balance and Balega Socks to arrange for GROW to receive more than one thousand pairs of their merchandise. To maximize outreach, GROW has arranged for school principals, social workers, teachers, coaches, and school resource deputies (sworn law enforcement officers) to request shoes for the students they serve.

GROW has also partnered with law enforcement staff to distribute a variety of sports balls to children and teens in low-income communities. In 2019, this program gave out 830 balls, including basketballs donated by Orlando Magic and soccer balls provided by the Orlando City Soccer Club and the Orlando Pride. GROW emblazoned many of the balls with empowering messages such as, "YOU GOT THIS," or "YOU ARE STRONG!" The balls also provide a vehicle for law enforcement officers to interact with youth in the community and help foster a positive relationship among these kids and trusted adult role models. The balls program thus serves as a vehicle for increasing physical activity, promoting social and emotional health, and supporting public safety all at the same time.

Thanks to cash and in-kind gifts from its supporters,

GROW provides other community services as well, including school playground renovations (with seven projects completed through 2019), donations of toys for school recess, and loans of materials for family-centered athletic events.

Challenges, Lessons, and Opportunities

The key to GROW's growth? According to Gonzalez, it's slowly and steadily building trust with schools, teachers, parents, and other community partners such as local businesses. A blessing and a curse of this process is the regular turnover among parents, whose kids graduate and move, and school administrators who retire or switch schools or jobs. New volunteers and principals need time to learn about GROW's work and how they can contribute to it, and then may be productive for only a couple of years before they are gone and the cycle begins anew. This means a constant loss of enthusiastic supporters and difficulty institutionalizing programs within schools, but it also provides an opportunity for a constant influx of new ideas and energy.

Another challenge: Almost all of the available donations from schools, volunteers, and even corporate partners are in-kind rather than monetary, requiring GROW to be especially resourceful. For example, GROW reminds schools to apply for grants that will cover the cost of items needed during the school year for running club or recess. GROW also facilitates collaboration among school PTAs and running clubs in hosting multi-school events, guiding them in what to expect and whom to call for help. To deliver needed supplies to schools efficiently and without direct cost, GROW has secured permission to use the school district's courier service. Gonzalez has also nurtured a culture of frugality among volunteers—for example, sharing equipment rather than buying it.

For Gonzalez, transitioning from doing everything herself to empowering other parents to lead activities has been a challenge but also a powerful opportunity. She marshalled her background in organizational behavior to recruit volunteers, to develop training materials and best practices, and to make it easy for parents to contribute to GROW's efforts without having to "reinvent the wheel" through trial and error. Increasingly, she sees GROW's mission as not just serving kids but also "taking parents that are green and teaching and developing them." In fact, GROW has become so successful as a volunteer-development organization that it now involves high school students as volunteer "action agents" who help promote community health through various projects and local events.

GROW Central Florida's accomplishments over the past 11 years have led to many trophies and awards, including the Seminole Association of School Administrators 2019–2020 Community Partner of the Year award, Florida Blue Foundation's 2017 Sapphire Award Recognizing Excellence and Innovation in Community Health, and Action for Healthy Kids' Healthy Hero Award and designation as a National Parent Ambassador. And the woman who started it all? Gonzalez was named one of *Orlando Magazine*'s 2020 Women of the Year.

Health Education Theory in Practice

Although GROW is neither academically designed nor evaluated, the organization's programs put into practice many important elements of health education theory.

For example, it has leveraged DOI (see chapter 5) by engaging with early adopters and thought leaders first while steadily building trust to enable a wider reach over time. Whereas at the beginning, Gonzalez needed to slowly build credibility for herself as an individual, the goodwill she enjoys now extends to GROW Central Florida as an organization. That, in turn, means that any new volunteer brought on does not need to start from scratch in terms of status; thanks to the organization's reputation, he or she can become trusted and productive quickly. Another DOI principle, that not all leaders are found in high places with the biggest titles, rings true for GROW. True to the "grass roots" in its name, GROW has focused on developing healthy children by mobilizing energy and willingness from the ground up.

GROW's work also applies SCT (see chapter 5) extensively. Its brand of teaching health is clearly not about telling but showing. Adult volunteers run with the kids, and officers play ball with them. This dynamic even extends to Gonzalez's interaction with parents. Through hands-on involvement, she not only models the skills needed to perform various tasks, but also provides moral authority by inspiring volunteers with a positive attitude and what she calls a "servant's heart." GROW supports environmental and social dimensions of health, both key components of behavior learning. It addresses the physical environment of health through distributing shoes and refurbishing playgrounds to make them more visually appealing, and the social environment of health by loaning equipment and offering technical assistance for family-centered events. Finally, GROW's work with student leaders adds a dimension of youth empowerment, which reinforces health behavior skills and attitudes by having kids demonstrate them to others.

The author would like to express his appreciation to Colleen Gonzalez's daughter, Morgan Gonzalez, an 18-year-old aspiring writer, for her valuable assistance in fact-checking and editing this case study. To learn more about GROW Central Florida, donate to support their work, or purchase activity equipment from their "wish list," visit www.growcentralflorida.org.

CHAPTER 6

SCHOOL CULTURE: KIDS VALUE WHAT WE DO, NOT WHAT WE SAY

What a school's social norms and attitude
about health communicate to students.

To make a real impact, schools will need to do a lot more than add SEL skill-building to their existing health class, if they even have one. According to SCT, behavior is developed through mastery of skills and observation of the lived—not spoken—values of the people we admire. And no one is better at identifying gaps between what we say and what we do than kids! So schools may need to change their own culture to prioritize health. For starters, consider the ways in which many schools show students that health education is really not that important.

Health Education Gets Bad Time

First and foremost, schools generally do not give health

education a prime-time slot. Health education tends to be filler, stuffed in around the unused edges of the schedule, borrowing shelf space from fine arts and music, placed in dead zones around holidays when everyone's mind is elsewhere, or cobbled into a short binge with an eye roll-worthy, euphemistic name like "Healthy Relationships Day" for sex ed. No wonder kids scoff at health education.

Health Education Gets Bad Timing

Another symptom of the disrespect schools show health education is that in many cases basic health concepts aren't taught until middle or high school. Nationwide, only half of elementary schools "require students to take classes that include instruction on health topics."[1] That portion rises to 68 percent among middle schools and 88 percent among high schools, but by then the attitudes, beliefs, and social norms that drive health behavior are more set and it may be too late to change them.[2,3]

The timing and nature of health education in the U.S. K–12 curriculum reflects several misperceptions, including:

1. Health education should revolve around warning of risks to be avoided, such as tobacco and alcohol, rather than promoting proactive behaviors such as exercise and nutrition.
2. Knowledge alone can prevent health problems.
3. Health knowledge and skills aren't needed until late middle or early high school.

The third one is an especially dangerous mindset because, by that point, health education may be coming after the risky behavior has started rather than before, when the education could have been preventive.

If we want to help kids develop better health behaviors that they can carry into adulthood, we need to make health education a fundamental part of early learning, building it into the educational foundation, like literacy and numeracy. Investing "upstream" in health education before teenage rebellion and experimentation set in can make healthy attitudes and behaviors automatic and reduce the "downstream" difficulty of fighting the health problem *du jour*, such as vaping (see chapter 7).

Health Education Teachers Aren't Empowered

Schools often delegate the responsibility of providing classroom health education to staff who are ill-equipped to do so. For example, making health education part of school health services is unrealistic and unfair to staff and students alike. (No offense to the few superstar nurses and counselors who provide both well.) If, as a nurse, your day is split between treating a child having an asthma attack, bandaging a bleeding knee, and planning a nutrition lesson, which of these activities will naturally get most of your time and priority? And how can we give the responsibility for health education to a counselor who is trained to handle discipline and behavior problems and to provide reactive, curative, one-on-one services—totally different skillsets from a classroom teacher's?

Sometimes health education is made the province of athletic coaches, who may not be trained in it or accountable for its results. They, or their school, may perceive that health education is a sideshow compared with their teams' win-loss record. That popular culture's latest caricature of a health teacher is the harsh and predatory Coach Carr in the movie *Mean Girls* is not only sad but also offensive and reveals the professional disrespect many physical educators and health educators contend with.

At some schools, any and all health education is combined with physical education. PE is too often an under-resourced department with low pay, a limited budget, and a higher-than-average student-teacher ratio, sometimes 50:1 or higher! In fact, 58 percent of schools report having no maximum student-teacher ratio for PE. To ask a teacher with no formal certification or training in health education to lead that instruction in a gym—much less with so many students at once, while also taking away from physical activity time—shows a clear lack of priority for this subject.

Finally, some schools abdicate health education completely and let outside (i.e., free) community health educators handle the load. Though highly knowledgeable, these experts possess no authority, meaning they also have no power to drive learning outcomes. When

I was a kid, whenever we had a substitute teacher, we unkindly all switched names and played dumb. As long as schools lack empowered and properly trained educators and pass health education around as a low-priority topic, we are throwing health to the wolves.

Physical Activity and Health Education Are Used as Punishment

Worse than providing unskilled instruction, many schools twist the teaching of health from a positive right granted to all students into a negative form of discipline forced on a few students. A meaningful number of schools (34 to 44 percent) permit physical activity to be withheld for poor behavior or incomplete classwork.[4] Some schools require tobacco prevention education only for students who are caught smoking or vaping. And 33 percent of schools allow the use of physical activity (e.g., running laps or doing push-ups) as a form of discipline, despite that doing so is considered corporal punishment and is therefore illegal in 29 states.[5,6] These approaches completely miss the point of prevention and harden anti-health attitudes among youth.

Health Education Lacks Accountability

Although many states include health education competencies within their stated learning standards, that does not mean health is taught and it certainly does not mean that health is tested. Schools greatly undermine health education through this absence of assessment and accountability for both teachers and students. Has a winning coach ever lost their job for poor health teaching? Health class is often optional, or taken for half-credit, or graded pass/fail, or not graded, or graded so leniently that anything below a B is the stuff of school-yard legend. In addition, health is not a subject on any required (or even optional) standardized test at any level of our K–12 educational system. Because school quality is measured to a large degree by students' performance on standardized tests, the absence of health questions on these tests also equates to a lack of accountability for schools themselves in the area of health education. Thus, schools' failure to prioritize health education is a simple reflection of their lack of incentives to do so.

Free and Inexpensive Solutions

So, what can schools who see value in health education—and want to demonstrate it through their actions—do within existing constraints of time and money?

First, recognize and leverage the powerful influence of "school attitude" (i.e., school leaders' attitudes, or "school culture") on student attitude and student behavior. School culture includes the social and environmental dimensions of SCT (see chapter 5) and shapes student behavior by demonstrating positive health beliefs and encouraging and rewarding students for holding those beliefs and performing healthy behaviors.

Second, take advantage of the fact that demonstrating

a positive school attitude toward health is, to a large degree, free. In many cases, adopting a healthy habit, vocabulary word, or policy takes no more time or money than an unhealthy one.

The CDC provides a list of no-cost best practices for teaching health including those mentioned below. The percentage of schools actually implementing each one is noted in parentheses.[7] Clearly, there is much room for progress without major investment.

- Require students who fail health class to retake it (26 percent).
- Provide lesson plans or learning activities to health educators (57 percent) and physical education teachers (46 percent).
- Devote health instruction time to health topics instead of combining it with physical education or another subject such as science (58 percent of middle and high schools; elementary schools rarely have health instruction time so were not surveyed).
- Offer regular physical activity breaks outside of PE (45 percent).
- Ensure that during PE students are moving most of the time rather than watching or waiting for their turn (71 percent).
- Prohibit or actively discourage food (including junk food) from being used "as a reward for good behavior or good academic performance" (47 percent).

To these I'll add: Replace sales of candy, sugared popcorn, or other unhealthy foods with healthy items like seasonal fruits or hold participatory fundraisers, such as physical activity challenges—they can raise as much or more money!

Solution: Walk the Walk

Schools should remember that we are always communicating, especially when surrounded by impressionable young minds. Look around you and notice examples of school leaders, staff, and parents communicating counterproductively about health behavior. Does the principal keep a candy bowl on the reception desk to "welcome" kids? Do teachers walk the halls holding sodas purchased in the faculty lounge while kids' beverages are limited to water and milk? Do parents refer to sugary drinks and processed snacks as "treats?" Do birthday parties and other events showcase sweet and fried foods? Since adults hone kids' attitudes and beliefs about health through role modeling, we need to adjust our conscious and unconscious communications to show that we value and celebrate healthy behavior, and most of all, that a healthy lifestyle is fun.

Principals, teachers, and parents can adopt simple habits such as noticing and remarking on kids' healthy behaviors—what we at CATCH call "CATCH Kids Being Healthy." For example, say to kids, "Looks like you tried the kale salad; it's good, isn't it?" or "You really kept moving out on the soccer field today!" And adults can model setting, sharing, and achieving their own health goals, such as walking two miles per day or eating one new vegetable per week. Kids need to learn to embrace health as a lifelong journey—one they can expect to include planning, hard work, setbacks, and successes.

Solution: Use the People and Time You Already Have

One perceived obstacle to better health education in schools is the lack of a specialized health teacher. While having one is certainly ideal and a worthy medium-term goal, almost all schools can improve health education with existing staff without overburdening them.

Since health is social, the environmental dimension of SEL-based health education is better delivered by a group than a single individual anyway. So, form a School Wellness Team. Teams incorporating existing personnel are more sustainable in the face of turnover, empower staff and students with important decision-making responsibility instead of placing it all in one pair of hands, and also model adult teamwork. The health leaders you are looking for are all around you, sometimes in the places you'd least expect. PE teachers and parent liaisons are obvious candidates, but also consider students, parents, executive assistants, classroom teachers, art teachers, librarians, administrators, and especially cafeteria staff (see chapter 9). Anyone who has positive health attitudes and behaviors and the ability to motivate others can become part of teaching health!

The idea of School Wellness Teams is certainly not new, but many are inactive. So, a school principal may need to inject a dose of motivation in the form of personal involvement, training, accountability, and/or a small monetary stipend. And simple gestures like public recognition for the team have a way of inducing action. I sometimes hear principals say that one of the best parts of creating a culture of health at their school is that it unites everyone in a winning cause and thus promotes more cohesion across the board.

When it comes to finding the time for health education, like anything in life, it's really a matter of priority and resourcefulness. Some schools use time in homeroom or advisory group meetings (one in New Orleans devotes the first 20 minutes of every Friday's homeroom to health lessons). Others integrate health lessons into science class; many use lunchtime to reinforce nutrition concepts. Just 40 minutes per week (24 hours per school year) of classroom time, not including physical activity time, provides an excellent dose of health education. But remember, no matter what the solution is for finding this time, to be effective, health teaching cannot follow a traditional facts-only method but needs to be accompanied by other components of SCT (see chapter 5).

Solution: Train the Team

As discussed, many of the teachers made responsible for health education—including the physical activity component—may not have a professional background in the subject, so they will need training. Even if they do have experience, they will need continuing education. Of course, training does take time and money, but often training a teacher to teach health can be done in place of training them in other topics they don't need, so it's an even trade. For example, it's a perennial complaint of physical educators that they have to endure mandatory trainings on topics like helping kids learn to read, instead of using that time for professional development that would be relevant to them.

Many school districts do have a head of health and PE (or "Whole Child"). This person may not be classified as a teacher but can invest in becoming a Master Certified Health Education Specialist through the National Committee for Health Education Credentialing and then provide free training to many teachers within their own school system. In addition to training, health educators need empowerment and moral, logistical, (and yes, financial) support from principals and district leaders if they are to succeed.

Solution: Test Health

Many educators and public health professionals complain that health education is destined to get short shrift because it's "not on the test." Well, there's an easy solution to that: let's put it on the test!

Schools are usually bound by a credit, testing, and grading system developed by their district or state, so principals and teachers may have limited latitude to take this action without support from higher up. If your school doesn't offer a graded health class, one way to get started is to include health education content in another course that *is* graded. Science is probably the most natural example, since many health concepts, such as the benefits of plant-based diets, and the importance of energy balance, relate to human physiology topics that are on the traditional menu. And since health is social, it can fit into social studies or language arts, too. Even math class can teach health; chapter 8's discussion on energy expenditure probably provides all the math you want in a day.

Schools or districts that wish to measure the impact of investing more in teaching health should measure a few key variables in a before-and-after fashion, including: overall academic performance, absenteeism, disciplinary cases, student knowledge of health, student attitudes and beliefs about health, self-reported student health behaviors, observational study of moderate-to-vigorous physical activity (MVPA) during activity time (see chapter 8), and student and parent perceptions of the value of health education. It can also be very revealing to teach one section of students more about health, and then ask them whether it was fun, interesting, and whether all students should be taught it.

Solution: Try It

Schools who are weighing the pros and cons of increasing the priority they place on teaching health should ask themselves: "What's the worst that can happen if we try?" Chapter 7 will explore an example of the worst that can happen if we don't try.

Summary

Because observational role modeling and environmental support are key parts of health behavior acquisition, our K–12 school system needs to *show* teachers and students that health education is important by allocating meaningful time for it and by providing the training, assessment, and accountability necessary for it to succeed. Schools can adopt many high-impact habits and practices without large investments of time or money.

Recommended Actions

Parents of school-age children: Ask your school and district how they train and support teaching health, whether by general teachers or specialists.

Teachers: Catch kids being healthy (i.e., practicing healthy behaviors and using health skills) and provide specific praise and positive reinforcement. Model healthy behavior, especially when you know students are watching.

Principals: Support the school health environment by making it a personal priority. Devote the same amount of time and attention to attending, observing, and evaluating School Wellness Team meetings, PE classes, and other health-related events and instruction that you give to reading and biology.

School boards, superintendents, and district administrators: "Put health on the test" by requiring and letter-grading 40 minutes per week of health education for every student (24 hours per school year).

Lawmakers and education policy makers: Add or update health education competencies in state learning standards. Put accountability behind them by adding health as a subject in state standardized tests across the K–12 spectrum and measuring performance.

CASE STUDY

District in Action—Goose Creek Consolidated Independent School District, Baytown, Texas

This school district in an industrial area outside Houston has seen tangible benefits from institutionalizing Whole Child health across all 21 of its elementary and junior high schools.

In 2014, MD Anderson Cancer Center received a significant gift from ExxonMobil, the largest company in the Baytown area, which operates the second-largest refinery in the U.S. there. This funding started the Be Well™ Baytown project, which began in 2017 and will be active through 2025 and supports implementation of a healthy-community model focused on modifiable cancer-risk factors. A major pillar of this cross-sector effort involves working with the local school district, Goose Creek CISD. Following the principles of Whole Child and the CDC's WSCC model (see chapter 3), the district sought to overhaul its health and wellness programming, with a focus on: physical education; nutrition; sun safety; staff wellness; coordination among nutrition services, health services, and related departments; parent and community involvement; and policies, systems, and environments conducive to wellness.

Planning

The planning process began when the Be Well Baytown team held high-level meetings to cultivate support for the multiyear project from the district superintendent, Dr. Randal O'Brien, and other school leaders. The district had already embraced the Whole Child philosophy—in fact, its mission statement is "Developing the Whole Child." As discussions progressed, it became clear that the CATCH program could help achieve the project's goals.

After the district had signed on in principle, Be Well Baytown funded a new position, Healthy Community School Coordinator, to serve as a champion of Whole Child health and wellness for the district. The district found the right person for the job among their very own ranks—Priscila Garza, a sixth-grade language arts teacher. One of her first tasks was to familiarize herself with CATCH and then develop an implementation plan for the district in coordination with the Be Well Baytown project team. Garza says that strong support for the program from their superintendent and other district leaders greatly smoothed the path of acceptance by principals and teachers—an important lesson for all districts that wish to increase the priority they place on teaching health.

A third crucial component of prelaunch planning was helping each participating school to build a diverse School Wellness Team (or "CATCH Team"), different from the Be Well Baytown project team, that included administrators, PE, and classroom teachers, nutrition services, and health services staff, and parents from that school. At about 70 percent of the schools, the team leader (or "CATCH Champion") is the PE teacher; a few other teams are led by administrators, such as an assistant principal, and one is even headed by an art teacher—further evidence that health advocates are all around us! As Garza notes, "One of the most effective parts of our program is bringing together teams of individuals that share a common goal of creating a culture of wellness in their school. Having a strong team of advocates is key in bringing awareness to any cause." (See chapter 6.) In addition to gaining internal support across the district, it was equally important to gain community support. Participating as the representative of one of the 23 community organizations that sit on Be Well Baytown's Steering Committee allowed Garza to foster relationships that helped the district in its effort to promote health and wellness.

Implementation

In its rollout plan, the district followed an important

principle of DOI (see chapter 5): To gain buy-in, begin with the thought leaders. So, for the first school year of its project (2017–2018), the district selected four pilot elementary schools that had particularly strong leadership and also stood to benefit the most. These schools served as demonstration models for future phases, while the participants provided continuous, real-world feedback on the program's rollout, and made recommendations for how to optimize it throughout the district.

Meanwhile, the district's 17 other elementary and middle schools began utilizing CATCH's physical education module only. This component was perceived to be the easiest to implement, since all schools already had a PE teacher and were adhering to the state-required minimum by providing 135 minutes of PE per child per week. The PE-only schools could thus focus on a single area of Whole Child health education—improving the quality of physical activity through higher moderate-to-vigorous intensity-level physical activity or MVPA (see chapter 8)—without needing to coordinate the efforts of multiple staff members. Moreover, their PE teachers could become familiar with CATCH's basic principles before implementing the program school-wide and leading or joining a School Wellness Team. Once the school rollout plan was set, the district trained all of the PE teachers and wellness teams on the CATCH program to provide them with the necessary knowledge, skills, and confidence to succeed. Garza also worked closely with each school to provide reinforcement training as needed and to address any challenges in implementation.

Beginning in the pilot period and continuing through-out its program rollout, Goose Creek applied the crucial social and environmental principles of SCT (see chapter 5) in two notable ways. First, in addition to CATCH program training, it provided staff training in the basic health knowledge they would be teaching as well as in personal wellness, which led to increased awareness of their own health behaviors. For example, staff reported that they became more conscious of the nutritional quality of their snacks and began to favor fruits and vegetables over junk foods, laying the groundwork for positive role modeling to kids. Second, the district's superintendent made personal appeals to teachers and principals to post stories, pictures, and videos about their school's health programming on official and personal social media. Ongoing communication and behavior modeling combined to build a self-reinforcing culture of health in the district, promoting the observational learning that is such an important part of teaching health.

Outcomes and Sustainability

The first three years of Goose Creek's CATCH program implementation across all 21 K–8 schools included accomplishments in three categories: process outcomes, health outcomes, and long-term sustainability.[1]

Process Outcomes

The district's process outcomes included:

- All schools promoted health messages such as GO-SLOW-WHOA in common areas; 50 percent of them used student work in that messaging.
- All schools held a Family Fun Event, with an average attendance of 170 people.
- 90 percent of schools communicated health tips to parents through PTA meetings or other official school channels.
- At least 80 percent of schools provided at least some in-classroom health teaching (this is not required in K-8, only high schools). Of those, half delivered the district-recommended dose of eight hours (12 class periods) per year and the other half provided approximately four hours per year.
- 70 percent of School Wellness Teams made presentations to their entire faculty on the Whole Child philosophy, CATCH's purpose, and available resources.

Taken together, these activities represent excellent progress in creating an environment of health, using communications that involve a wide variety of stakeholders and orienting health activities toward celebration and fun (see chapter 9).

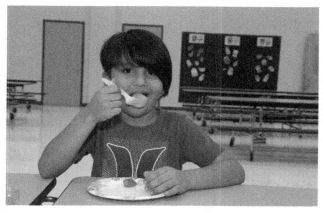

A Goose Creek CISD student enjoys seasonal fruits (note kid-made nutrition education mural in background) (Photograph by Goose Creek CISD. Used with permission.)

Health Outcomes

District students also benefitted from these key health outcomes:

- Children reported eating more healthy foods, including a 33 percent increase in the number of servings of vegetables they consumed.
- Children reported drinking 12 percent more water.
- Independent, trained evaluators found a 27 percent increase in the portion of PE class kids spent in MVPA (from 45 percent to 57 percent). This represents a progression from 10 percent below the CDC recommendation to 14 percent above it (see figure 6 and chapter 8).

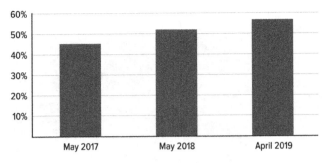

Figure 6: Portion of PE Class Time Goose Creek CISD Students Spent in Moderate-to-Vigorous Physical Activity (MVPA)

Sustainability

A key metric for CATCH and related Whole Child initiatives is the extent to which they are "institutionalized;" that is, built into the budget and a routine part of the district's ongoing work, rather than being short-term or worse, one person's pet project. Schools run on annual calendars and other routines, so securing a place for teaching health in that cycle is often the hardest part. Another important component of sustainability is succession. For example, what happens when a school's Wellness Champion leaves? This happened at Goose Creek six times in three years. In most cases, another member of the Wellness Team stepped into the leadership position. In one case, when an administrator was reassigned to a new school, the principal simply told their replacement that they would be leading the Wellness Team—that role was now part of the administrator's job description. In another instance, the Champion went on maternity leave and an assistant principal (who had been on a Wellness Team at another school) stepped up to serve on an interim basis. Thus, different schools came up with different plans, but all established precedents for ensuring succession. None left the Wellness Team without a leader, even temporarily, or asked meekly for volunteers, or kicked the vacancy down the road to be dealt with another day—as too often happens in organizations of all types!

Another means of institutionalizing Whole Child wellness is by building its expenses into the district's budget. Be Well Baytown covered all costs associated with implementing the program for the first three school years (2017–2018 through 2019–2020). Over the next three (2020–2021 through 2022–2023), the district will move toward self-sustainability by progressively taking over from Be Well Baytown the $120,000 per year cost of maintaining the program infrastructure. With almost 25,000 students in the district, this amount works out to under $5 per child per year—less than the cost of a single lunch!

The largest component of this investment goes to employing the district's Healthy Community Schools Coordinator, initially Garza, who serves as a trainer and coach for each School Wellness Team and advocates for the program to district administrators and principals. All of the rest of the work involved in running the programs is built into the job descriptions of existing staff. Although an ideal culture makes participation in teaching health a small part of every teacher and administrator's job requirements, it is unrealistic to expect it to be a major part of a superintendent or principal's day. Even with excellent institutionalization, Whole Child health, like all programs, requires ongoing training, oversight, and adaptation. Having at least one professional to orchestrate it across a district is indispensable.

Plans for Continued Improvement

As Goose Creek CISD looks ahead to its next round of progress in teaching health, it sees three initiatives on the horizon. First, and most important, is continuing to expand classroom health education. With a dedicated health class only available and required in high school, Goose Creek's Program Coordinator hopes to work with the district's Curriculum Specialists, or "Content Coordinators," for each subject to identify courses into which health topics can be incorporated. Garza points out that science is the most obvious subject—a unit on anatomy could include learning how the body uses vitamins and nutrients commonly found in plants and how the heart muscle is strengthened by exercise, thus improving blood flow and delivering oxygen to the brain. Language arts is another area where health-related material can be included—for example, in reading assignments. The district also seeks to integrate health with its SEL program, which includes developing positive social attitudes and making responsible health-behavior decisions.

A second goal is having all schools continually maintain and improve the CATCH Whole Child program as part of their Campus Improvement Plan. (Texas requires all schools to have such a plan to qualify for funding under the federal Every Student Succeeds Act, the law that replaced No Child Left Behind.) According to Garza, "Some principals already highlight Whole Child efforts in their plans as an opportunity to showcase their schools, but there is not yet a requirement that they do so, nor accountability for those who do not."

Finally, the district plans to bolster the effectiveness of its School Health Advisory Council (SHAC), a state-mandated body that oversees all health-related activities in a district's schools. Around Texas, some SHACs are very active, while others barely exist due to a lack of enforcement. Beginning with the 2020–2021 school year, Goose Creek CISD will place management of its SHAC under its Healthy Community School Coordinator, who will focus on involving more senior school leaders and community members, and organizing more frequent meetings of the council.

Summary

Goose Creek CISD has traveled a long way in improving Whole Child programming and teaching health through:

1. cultivating strong support from the district superintendent and board-level leadership
2. employing a full-time coordinator and institutionalizing routines for training teachers, sustaining principal support, and maintaining active wellness teams at the large majority of district schools

3. creating a reporting infrastructure that steadily increases accountability
4. developing a sustainability plan around this vitally important educational mission.

Their work provides an excellent example of what can be done by a school district to organize and standardize the teaching of health in all of its schools.

ACTIVITY BREAK

My Bonnie Lies over the Ocean

Let's take a break and keep learning fun and productive!

Exercise enhances learning by stimulating the brain. We are more effective teachers when we show rather than merely tell what we want students to learn (see chapter 5). So, this may be the first book you ever read that incorporates a physical activity break. Before you roll your eyes, remind yourself that activity helps you think better.

Now stand up, step away from your chair into a clear space, and let's go!

In your head or out loud, you are going to sing the classic song, "My Bonnie Lies over the Ocean." On each "B" sound, do a squat by *bending* your knees as far as you can while facing forward and keeping your back upright. Modify the move to suit your physical condition, but don't cheat by going too easy on yourself.

My Bonnie lies over the ocean.
My Bonnie lies over the sea.
My Bonnie lies over the ocean.
Oh, bring back my Bonnie to me.

Bring back, bring back
Oh, bring back my Bonnie to me, to me.

Bring back, bring back
Oh, bring back my Bonnie to me!
[applause and bow]

PART III

HOW?

TEACHING FOUNDATIONAL HEALTH BEHAVIORS

CHAPTER 7

TOBACCO AVOIDANCE: DEFUSING THE E-CIGARETTE EXPLOSION

*How the epidemic of youth vaping happened
and how health education can mitigate it.*

Q: What could possibly go wrong if we don't take K–12 health education seriously?

A: The youth vaping epidemic.

As of the summer of 2020, the crisis of youth electronic-cigarette use, or vaping, is still in full flame. Though a full post-mortem is premature, we are far enough along to examine how it started and to consider the role health education could have played in limiting its spread—and can still play in its eventual control and decline.

Where We Are and Why That's a Problem

The National Youth Tobacco Survey conducted by the FDA and CDC concluded that in 2019, 5.4 million middle and high schoolers "currently" used e-cigarettes (i.e., during the past 30 days).[1] That's a staggering two-and-a-half-fold increase from 2017.

The health dangers to kids of typical e-cigarettes include addiction to nicotine, potential harm to brain development, and the unknown long-term health impacts of inhaling the other chemicals the product contains. I say "typical" because for a while, e-cigarettes and vaping were synonymous mainly with the delivery of nicotine, but vaping has come to encompass inhaling controlled substances such as THC and CBD along with many other chemicals that can be aerosolized. So, although vaping is really a behavior and not a specific drug, we will focus on nicotine since most school-age vapers use mass-market e-cigarettes that contain it (including all JUULs, their favorite brand until recent changes in law, described below).

Nicotine is uniquely dangerous to youth because the further a child's brain is from reaching full development at around age 26, the more susceptible that child is to becoming addicted to it—almost 90 percent of adult tobacco users took up the habit by age 18, and 99 percent by age 26.[2] This fact should make everyone skeptical of claims from the nicotine-delivery industry that they don't want youth using their products. Without addicting youth, simple math tells us that their business can't continue beyond a generation or two.

The *Surgeon General's Advisory on E-cigarette Use Among Youth* warns that, in addition to being addictive, nicotine can cause reduced impulse control, mood disorders, and attention and cognition deficits in youth.[3] Would any parents or teachers like to have their teens use a product that would give them *lower* impulse control, *more* mood disorders, and *less* attention and cognition?

Vaping also carries several other health, social, and educational risks for youth:

- Youth who vape are almost seven times more likely to start smoking cigarettes within 18 months than those who don't.[4]
- People addicted to nicotine are more likely to become addicted to other drugs, both illicit and prescription.[5,6]
- Vaping is detrimental to immune health and lung function,[7] and therefore it is biologically plausible that vaping is a risk factor for getting COVID-19, and if you do get it, having a more severe case. (As of this writing, this risk has been demonstrated for smoking and is suspected for vaping.[8])
- Manufactured e-cigarettes contain many chemical compounds with unknown short- and long-term health effects. Perhaps worse, refillable vaping devices have inspired home-brew experimentation that is minimally regulated—besides nicotine, youth vape THC, CBD, and other concoctions. An outbreak of E-cigarette and Vaping Associated Lung Injury (EVALI) in late 2019 harmed more than 2,800

people and was ultimately traced to Vitamin E acetate, a thickening agent added to vaping products containing THC.[9] EVALI may be only the first of many vaping-related diseases to come.

- Although vaping is less expensive than smoking, it is still not cheap. At 2020 prices, a $4.00 JUUL pod contains the same amount of nicotine as a pack of cigarettes, which costs an average of $7.00. This expense may distort youth behavior and lead to crime. An Austin-area high schooler was murdered in 2019 in a presumed vaping sale stick-up,[10] and teens are routinely caught shoplifting e-cigarette pods and devices, sometimes leading to a criminal record for life.

- The more normalized youth vaping becomes, the greater the negative social consequences for those who don't participate, including bullying and exclusion.

- Vaping is a giant distraction from education because kids leave class to feed their addiction, sneak a hit right in the classroom when the teacher isn't looking, miss school due to suspension, or are otherwise unable to properly concentrate on learning.

Considering the well-known dangers of tobacco and the hard-won social norms disfavoring its use, how is it possible that it could be so quickly repackaged and revisited upon our youth with such grotesque success? A proper answer to this question must address both the supply side (the product and its availability) and the demand side (how youth feel about its use).

How We Got Here: Supply Side

E-cigarettes were introduced around 2007 as a potentially safer alternative to cigarettes. Like smoking cigarettes, e-cigarette use involves inhaling from a handheld device to deliver nicotine through the lungs and into the bloodstream. And because nicotine comes from the tobacco plant, e-cigarettes are considered tobacco products. However, whereas smoking involves burning tobacco leaves and therefore inhaling the many carcinogenic by-products of combustion, using e-cigarettes involves heating a nicotine-containing fluid into a "vapor" or aerosol that is *probably* less harmful than tobacco smoke. (If it isn't obvious why that is faint praise, see more in the health education section below.)

E-cigarettes have evolved into three product categories, each of which has different effects on and appeals to youth. They are listed below in order of their appearance on the market:

1. Disposables. These were the first e-cigarettes on the market and are typically of the same size and shape as traditional cigarettes. Initially they were not offered in exotic flavors, and their appeal was mostly limited to adults trying to reduce the harm of their nicotine use while still having an experience similar to smoking. Youth dismissed them as being "for old people." Unfortunately, following the 2020 rules limiting flavors of pre-filled e-cigarettes (see below), many flavored disposables have appeared and youth have been drawn in.

2. Refillables. Also known as "pens," "tanks," or "mods," these e-cigarettes are larger and usually held in the palm of the hand instead of between two fingers. As their name suggests, these devices allow repeated use with "e-juice" (the suspension of nicotine in an easily aerosolized propellant) available in lightly regulated neighborhood vape shops all over the country. The advent of these devices has led to a proliferation of vape flavors: hot cinnamon, sour apple, crème brûlée, Dr. Pepper, cotton candy, pancakes and maple syrup, spearmint, T-bone steak, unicorn vomit (no kidding, Google it)—or if none of those sound tempting enough, any one of about eight thousand other varieties. These products first gained popularity with young adults and were generally too expensive, cumbersome, and messy to take off with middle- and high-schoolers (who labeled them "douche flutes"). The biggest niche for these devices in the youth market today is for vaping THC or CBD.

3. Pre-filled. This type of device contains a snap-in "cartridge" or "pod" containing flavored e-juice. The most notable example is JUUL, which burst on the scene in 2017 and in less than three years, vastly expanded the under-18 market for vaping and captured 75 percent of it.[11] Sometimes called the "iPhone of e-cigarettes," JUUL resembles a flash drive and is thus both sleeker and easier to conceal than other devices. With a smaller range of flavors and pre-filled pods, its simpler packaging made it

much easier to stock and sell than other types of vaping devices. When JUUL appeared, many teens were suddenly able to get e-cigarettes by faking their age and ordering online, finding a corner store or gas station with lax age enforcement, or locating an enterprising friend who had bought in quantity (legally or illegally) and would resell to them. Finally, JUUL's breakthrough in using "nicotine salts" allowed it to make a higher-nicotine product, which it trumpeted delivered nicotine to the brain 1.25 to 2.7 times faster than other e-cigarettes.[12] JUUL's innovative combination of being appealing, accessible, addictive, and discreet led to its adoption by millions of K–12 students around the country.

Regulatory Response

The vaping crisis has triggered a new era of tobacco regulation. However, a fierce tug-of-war persists between those who point to the potential harm-reduction of vaping compared with use of other tobacco products and those who point to the soaring popularity of vaping products among youth and their health risks, both known and unknown.

To address the youth accessibility side of the equation, on December 20, 2019, President Donald Trump signed a law setting the minimum age to purchase any tobacco product at 21 years old. This change followed decades of advocacy and was undoubtedly spurred by the escalation of youth vaping and the enactment of similar laws in 19 states, including six of the seven most populous, in the years leading up to it.

In terms of youth appeal, many public health advocates have raised alarms that 81 percent of youth ages 12–17 report that their first experience with tobacco was with a flavored product (possibly because flavors mask the natural bitterness of nicotine and thus lower the barrier to initiation).[13] It seemed clear that despite e-cigarettes' promise of reducing harm to existing tobacco users, their exotic and sweet flavoring was creating harm by attracting young newcomers.

Thus, in September 2019, the Trump administration suggested a "flavor ban" on all e-cigarettes. After several months of intense lobbying by the vaping industry, the new rules that took effect in February 2020 only limit flavors in "pre-filled" cartridge devices. Menthol and tobacco flavors are exempt from restrictions across all devices. Initial reports suggest that since the change, youth e-cigarette use has simply shifted to the other two device types (disposables and tanks), which have fewer or no flavor restrictions.

Other innovations have quickly sprung up as well. For example, Puff Krush, whose marketers describe it as "pre-filled [flavor] pods designed to be an add-on for the [tobacco] JUUL pod."[14] Krush pods are exempt from regulation because they contain no nicotine. So, by simply separating the nicotine and the flavoring into two different packages, manufacturers circumvented the regulations in less time than it took to make them. In summary, the flavor ban did not turn out to be a flavor ban at all.

How We Got Here: Demand Side

Since it takes two to tango, we also need to consider why today's youth have been so uniquely susceptible to vaping.

First, their teachers and parents didn't grow up with JUULs or other e-cigarettes and simply don't have the life experience, facts, or vocabulary at hand to confidently discuss and bust myths about them. (What life experience we parents *do* have strongly argues for not taking up topics with our teens that we have not mastered ourselves!) So, most young people have not received the basic social inoculation against the dangers of e-cigarettes that they have against traditional cigarettes, marijuana, other drugs, drunk driving, unprotected sex, and other common youth health risks.

This yawning generational knowledge gap was unmistakable to me when I brought a JUUL to the largest annual gathering of high-school future health professionals (HOSA) in the summer of 2018, after this product had already been around for a while. Of the five hundred or so adults I presented to, only two or three hands went up when I asked what it was. Meanwhile, my colleagues and I were unsuccessful in finding a single high schooler among the thousands in attendance with any such uncertainty. We did, however, collect a few classic "Duh!" looks along the way.

The second compounding element of this perfect storm was the advent of social media and micro-marketing, which allowed kids to be targeted with messages their parents weren't seeing at all. If e-cigarette makers had taken out ads in *TIME* magazine like tobacco peddlers of yore, adults would have cottoned to the dangers quickly and the period of parental cluelessness about vaping would have been much shorter. Instead, e-cigarette manufacturers, especially JUUL, exploited channels unmonitored by grown-ups through the use of paid social media "influencers" on Twitter, Instagram, and YouTube. These influencers' posts portray the product as cool and evoke emotions such as relaxation, freedom, and sex appeal. Often including images of youth, they easily reached underage consumers.

A third reason that parents and teachers were caught unawares is, ironically, that youth smoking prevention policies and programs—including hard-hitting youth awareness media campaigns like those from the non-profit Truth Initiative—were so successful. From the mid-1990s to 2018, the portion of eighth-to-twelfth graders smoking cigarettes on a daily basis plunged 88 percent.[15] Perhaps it is only natural that parents and schools shifted their attention away from teen nicotine use. But in so doing, we left our kids unguarded from the predations of Big Tobacco and e-cigarette upstarts like JUUL. And when they hit, those decades of neglect of health education meant schools were without the staff skill, schedule time, parent engagement, and culture of teaching health needed to mount a rapid response.

How Health Education Can Help

The dizzying rise of youth vaping shows that when it comes to health education, parents can't keep up, and because they don't make it a core priority, schools don't keep up. Skills-based health education that applies SCT and SEL could have helped stop the march of the vaping epidemic—and still can, in three ways.

The first is by disseminating knowledge through posters and other environmental supports in schools, as well as through classroom education that includes account-ability measured through assignments and tests. Just because youth are familiar with vaping does not mean they understand it, and in the absence of formal (or at least parental) health education, teens bear the weight of dangerous myths passed peer-to-peer. For example, 59 percent of youth think e-juice is mostly water (it actually has none) and 41 percent think that if e-cigarettes are fla-vored, it means they don't contain nicotine (99 percent of mass-market products and all JUULs do).[16,17] This latter myth was passively stoked by the industry, which did not clearly label their products as containing nicotine until required to do so in August 2018.[18] In an illustration of our youths' own anger at the lack of information about vaping available to them, a number of youth-initiated lawsuits have been mounted alleging that manufacturers intentionally deceived the public about e-cigarettes' nicotine content.

The second benefit health education could provide is to cultivate healthy attitudes and beliefs about e-cigarettes. Many youths, to some extent abetted by adults, have underrated the dangers of vaping due to whatever is the opposite of "guilt by association" with cigarettes. Let's call it "innocence by dissociation." School-age youth mostly still harbor social antibodies against smoking combustible tobacco but see vaping as fundamentally different, rather than as the same old drug (nicotine) delivered in a different package. No wonder, since e-cigarettes have been promoted as a potentially safer alternative to cigarettes. In fact, JUUL illegally said "safer" until September 2019, when it received a harsh cease-and-desist letter from the FDA on that subject.[19]

Anyway, "potentially safer" is hardly consolation when you are comparing something with an unquantified risk with one of the deadliest products of all time. Used as designed, cigarettes have already caused one hundred million deaths and add another one hundred planeloads of fatalities every day.[20] And there's certainly no need for a "safer alternative" for the millions of kids who never smoked in the first place! A good health teacher can guide youth to reframe unhealthy beliefs (for example, changing "this is safer" to "safer is not safe"), and in so doing significantly improve health behaviors.

Finally, health education can combat demand for vaping

through youth empowerment. It's pretty clear that the dogmatic "just say no" approach never worked, and it certainly doesn't work with today's teens.[21] Instead, teachers need to help kids make their own decisions about health behaviors and arm them with the social skills to back them up. For example:

- Instead of asking students to make a "pledge" not to vape, ask them to make a "choice" about vaping. Pledges can feel coerced and, like forced apologies, may not be sincere. Making a choice is much more empowering.
- Rather than making declarative statements, ask open-ended questions about how vaping could hinder kids' own goals. This helps them to reflect and formulate connections in their own minds between their behaviors and the short- and long-term consequences of those actions.
- As part of the health curriculum, organize peer-led small-group discussions and report-outs facilitated by peer-elected leaders. This format helps youth hear health messages in their peers' own words and promotes participation and candor.
- Guide youth in naming and practicing peer-refusal skills. Rehearsing refusal is crucial because the moment when (not if) a child is offered an e-cigarette may well be in a socially charged atmosphere where there is little time to formulate a confident reply.
- Provide project-based learning opportunities for teens to explain, share, and advocate publicly for their healthy choice through presentations, posters,

PSA videos, and social media. This evangelism will help cement their decision and beliefs into their own identity while potentially persuading some of their peers to follow their lead (see case study on "Student in Action" following this chapter).

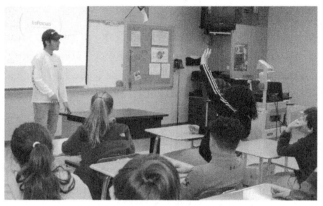

High schooler Luka Kinard speaks about vaping to a class of peers at Hickory High School, North Carolina (Photograph by Beverly Snowden, Director of Communications, Hickory Public Schools. Used with permission.)

These techniques help develop healthy attitudes and empowering skills, particularly important in combatting the billions of dollars in advertising poured into making vaping look cool. If health educators are going to help kids replace marketers' hollow emotional appeals with an attitude that it's health that is cool, a facts-only, adult-delivered approach will not work. The strongest and most durable health behaviors are the ones cultivated by training youth to think and act for themselves.

Pitfalls to Avoid

In addition to following these best practices, schools that want to make an impact on student vaping through health education will need to break a few bad habits.

First, resist the temptation to plug the topic of vaping into an already weak approach to school health education. Schools need to acknowledge when they're behind and actively remediate the problem. I have attended several presentations for parents in which a school triumphantly announced that vaping will be added as a topic in the (one-and-done) sixth-grade health class next year! Invariably, an irate parent will raise their hand and say, "What about my seventh grader who will be in eighth grade next year—what are you doing for her?" And if no one is saying it, they're still thinking it. If you are the one fielding that question, how will you reply?

Second, don't limit vaping education to students who are caught in the act. Quality youth health education programs reform some kids, but their strength is in prevention, not treatment. And for a bona fide addict, the remedy may need to go beyond education to therapy with counseling and/or medication.

Moreover, making health education a punishment is a bad precedent and a huge disservice to kids who, with a dose of prevention, might have avoided an infraction in the first place. Assigning kids a community-service project like making an anti-vaping poster or video may be an instructive disciplinary "learning experience," but it's no substitute for making vaping prevention part of the educational core.

And finally, don't let up when this particular crisis passes. Being a good educator means staying at the forefront of new information and trends. As the vaping epidemic has amply illustrated, health education topics and techniques evolve at least as fast as those of any other subject. Health needs to be made a part of schools' educational core once and for all so that when the next threat emerges, we are in front of it rather than playing catch-up with a generation of children.

Summary

The epidemic of youth vaping was caused by the combination of rapidly evolving and poorly regulated repackaging of nicotine (supply side) and a vacuum of adult awareness and school health education (demand side). Educationally sound and up-to-date approaches to health behavior skill-building and youth empowerment have been shown to help reduce vaping among K–12 students, but to make meaningful progress, more schools need to reform poor health education habits.

Recommended Actions

Teachers and parents of school-age children: Inform yourself about vaping basics and ask your school how they are addressing the epidemic.

Principals: Provide youth vaping-prevention education proactively, rather than as a disciplinary response. Host a required informational session for staff and an optional one for parents.

School boards, superintendents, and district administrators: Require evidence-based vaping prevention education for all students in grades five through twelve. (Although some experts advocate starting even sooner, others claim that can backfire by kindling curiosity.) View the vaping epidemic as a symptom of a chronic lack of health education in schools, not an isolated problem to be overcome and forgotten.

CASE STUDY

Student in Action—Romi Eldah, Avon High School Class of 2020, Avon, Connecticut

During Romi Eldah's senior year at Avon High School, he undertook a vaping- prevention project that won the gold medal in the inaugural CATCH My Breath Service Learning Project competition. Along with a $2,500 college scholarship, Romi received a perfect score of 60/60 from the expert judging panel—and when you read this case study, you'll understand why. Rather than paraphrase his story, I will let Romi tell it himself through these lightly edited direct quotes compiled from his contest application.

Origin and Purpose

As a student athlete, my health and wellness have been important to me my whole life. At my school, I'm required to complete a Senior Mastery Capstone Project before I graduate, so I chose to research the effects of vaping and the impact it has on the health of today's youth. Although I've always done my best to discourage kids from vaping, my warnings about the potential harm they were doing to their bodies with every inhalation were often ignored. I just didn't have the impact I had hoped to have, so I decided to learn more about this growing epidemic and figure out how I could make a difference here in my community. My goals were to complete three different service projects: deliver a great Capstone community presentation, bring the CATCH My Breath Program to Avon High School, and create a fundraising project for the cause.

Capstone Presentation

First, I met with my anatomy teacher, Jessie Shaw, about the topic of vaping and its health effects on today's youth to ask her if she thought it was a good topic for Capstone, and if she would be my mentor and advisor. She was interested and agreed.

The topics I researched for my presentation included an overview of vaping, statistics on the rise in vaping use, marketing strategies targeting youth, chemical dangers, impact on health, and potential risks to body systems, addiction concerns, and vaping as a possible gateway to other drugs, how we can help make a difference in our community, the CATCH My Breath Program, and local, state, and federal laws around vaping.

As with any presentation, I prepared and practiced long

and hard to perfect each element. I was a week or two away from my presentation date when the coronavirus surprised us all and knocked me off my well-planned path. We moved to remote learning, so I was forced to leave my comfort zone and do something I had never done before. I had to present my Capstone over Zoom to my mentor and a grading panel of teachers while my family was there watching me.

When it was finally time to present, I was a nervous wreck, trying to make small talk before my presentation as I tested the angle of the monitor, the camera, my links, and more. My mentor mentioned that how I was feeling was just what she felt when the teachers began teaching remotely. What was amazing, though, is that once I began my presentation, my nerves washed away. I dialed in and knocked it out of the park. I passed "with distinction," having gone "above and beyond" what was required, and I will be recognized for my hard work and exceptional results.

Bringing CATCH My Breath to Avon High School

When I was doing the vaping research for my Capstone Project, I found information about the CATCH My Breath Program online. I was really interested in the idea of bringing the program to my school. The website was informative, and I also was able to speak with someone in the office directly about the different service-learning projects that were offered by CATCH My Breath.

After talking with the assistant principals, I was able to meet with my high school principal, Michael Renkawitz. I knew my principal was very busy and that I might only have one chance at impressing him and getting my point through. So I prepared my notes about why I wanted to bring a vaping prevention program to our school, what it meant to me, and why it was important to our entire school. I explained the details of how the CATCH My Breath school program works and gave him the CATCH brochure and their website address. I also informed him about how successful their program is by sharing their research, which says that seven out of eight students say they are less likely to use e-cigarettes after CATCH My Breath. We agreed to set up another meeting after he'd reviewed the information. Unfortunately, due to COVID-19, we just didn't have time to finalize the plan. Instead of meeting in person, we had to move to communicating remotely through email.

Fortunately, I did achieve my goal and he agreed to join the movement, stating "Avon High School has officially joined the CATCH My Breath Program; doing so gives us access to the researched student presentations, short lessons, parent information, and future updates." He indicated that he was proud of what I had done in representing Avon High School's student body, and that I was helping our community as a whole.

Although we were faced with the obstacle of COVID-19 and were not able to deliver the program this spring, it will begin in the fall. I will be in college then, but look forward to hearing all about it from my younger brother. I am glad I persevered and didn't let COVID-19 derail the plan, and I hope that Avon High School is able to offer this program for many, many years. It will be a great resource for the parents, teachers, and school staff who work so hard to support the health and education of children and students.

Fundraising Project

I met with the principal a second time to talk about my idea to sell custom bracelets that I had designed with the message "HEALTH IS YOUR WEALTH, DON'T GET SUCKED IN" at school. We discussed how donations to the CATCH My Breath Program support vaping prevention education in schools and that for every $25 raised, 50 students could be educated. During this meeting, I was given permission to sell custom bracelets as a fundraiser. We decided on a time and location for me to sell them; for example, during our lunch break as everyone was walking to the cafeteria.

Unfortunately, the coronavirus forced me to find another way to sell them, so I turned to social media, posting stories on my Instagram and Snapchat as well as messaging my friends, teammates, neighbors, and relatives. I had countless responses saying how great the idea was and that I was doing an amazing thing. I couldn't believe the support I received.

Knowing I had to keep to social-distancing rules, I

collected addresses, drove the bracelets to drop off in people's mailboxes, and picked up the donations they had left for me. I included an insert explaining that $25 of donations reaches 50 students and that there was new research being done to address the links between vaping and infectious diseases like COVID-19.

This fundraiser reached 100 percent of my goal of raising $250, allowing me to help CATCH My Breath provide vaping prevention education to over five hundred students!

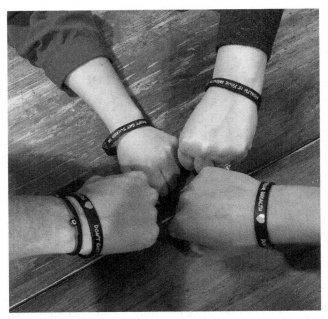

Romi Eldah's promotional picture of his anti-vaping bracelets (Photograph by Romi Eldah. Used with permission.)

Conclusions and Lessons Learned

I estimate I have spent more than two hundred hours working on my Capstone and these service projects over more than six months. I certainly benefited a lot from learning and studying this topic and feel like I can now better teach others to help prevent them from starting to use e-cigarettes or encourage those who are already using to stop. I have a much better understanding about the vaping epidemic and addiction, the effects of vaping on the human body, how it can affect the health of today's youth, and how important it is to offer vaping-prevention education.

These projects also helped me develop important life skills I will use next year in college and hopefully for years after, like how to thoroughly research and present on a topic that I am passionate about to a group, whether in person or remotely using Zoom. I went from being nervous with the idea of public speaking to actually enjoying it. I also benefited a lot through the fundraising process of designing and selling my bracelets. I learned how to reach out to people to ask them to support a cause by educating them and being sure they knew how their donation would be used to make a difference. It taught me how to advocate for something I believed in and how to find different ways to spread awareness and get my message out.

Now that my high school is officially part of the CATCH My Breath Program, I see that I can make a difference with causes that are important to me and can be successful if I'm willing to put in the hard work and stay focused on the goal. And with the unprecedented times of COVID-19, not only did I learn how to be flexible and adaptable, but I now know that you have to be persistent and determined to find ways to reach your goal even when things don't go as planned.

My plan for the fall is to attend Springfield College in their Master of Science Physician Assistant Studies Program. Being awarded a scholarship from CATCH My Breath would be such a huge help for me, as I would put it toward paying for my education. I plan to continue to spread the word about the dangers of vaping and remind people that "HEALTH IS YOUR WEALTH, DON'T GET SUCKED IN."

Congratulations on your service to your peers and community, Romi! And thank you for allowing me to share your work in this book. Kudos also go to the team at Avon High School who, by supporting Romi, demonstrated the principles of youth empowerment so important to the effective teaching of health (see chapter 9).

CHAPTER 8

PHYSICAL ACTIVITY: MAXIMIZING THE TIME WE ALREADY HAVE

A solution for overloaded school schedules: Increasing exercise intensity offers the same aerobic benefits as adding more time for physical activity.

Note: The terms Physical Education (PE) and Physical Activity (PA) overlap; the main difference is that PE focuses on movement-oriented physical skill-building, whereas PA focuses on movement itself. Sometimes the term "structured PA" is used to distinguish adult-supervised activities that require movement from "recess," when movement is optional. Since research demonstrates a correlation between PA and both health and educational benefits, we'll use the term PA here.

Fighting for Minutes

How many minutes of the school day or week should

be devoted to PA is a hotly debated topic, and one with a zero-sum mentality. Each minute added to the quota is perceived as a gain for health advocates but a loss for educators, and vice versa for each minute subtracted. Parents can be found on both sides of the debate.

For example, the California Education Code requires all elementary schools to provide two hundred minutes of PA to students every 10 school days. Frustrated with a 50 percent compliance rate, along with independent findings that the rule was rarely enforced, in 2013 San Francisco-area elementary school parent, Marc Babin, and his advocacy group Cal200 sued 37 districts around the state.[1]

A Hollow Victory?

Cal200 eventually won, but the newly enforced minutes of PA in California can be supervised by anyone with a state teaching certification. In other words, teachers are required to lead PA but are not required to have any experience or professional development in doing so. Naturally, many teachers who suddenly find themselves needing to cover PA are at a loss for how to teach it, and one can hardly expect them to do so without formal training. To understand why this outcome makes Cal200's case less of a victory than it seems requires understanding how PA is measured and the amount of exercise children need for a beneficial health effect.

The Measure That Really Matters

The scientific unit of measure for PA is MET-minutes, movement time (in minutes) multiplied by movement intensity (in Metabolic Equivalents, or METs). A MET is the ratio of oxygen consumed when moving compared with oxygen consumed at rest. Oxygen consumption at rest is the baseline and has a MET of 1.0. Physical activity with an intensity of less than 3.0 METs—which means you're exerting less than three times the energy you would sitting still—is classified as light, 3.0–5.9 METs is considered moderate, and 6.0 or more METs is considered vigorous.

For protection against cancer and other noncommunicable diseases, the U.S. Department of Health and Human Services (HHS) recommends a PA "dose" of 500–1,000 MET-minutes per week for average adults.[2] Based on the 2011 Compendium of Physical Activities, which lists hundreds of activities and their MET levels, this recommendation could be met by, for example, running at six mph for 25 minutes three times a week:

> 25 minutes of movement time x 9.8 METs = 245 MET-minutes x 3 days = 735 MET-minutes.

It could also be met by raking a lawn for four hours a week:

> 240 minutes x 4.0 METs = 960 MET-minutes.[3]

Health agencies sometimes simplify their PA guidelines

by expressing them in minutes, and therefore that is how many people think of them. For example, many adults consider a good exercise goal to be 20 minutes per day, 5 days per week (100 minutes per week). But as shown in the examples above and in figure 7, minutes of exercise mean little without considering intensity. Doing 100 minutes of physical activity per week at an intensity of 3.0 METs is not enough; 100 minutes at 6.0 METs is near the bottom of the recommended range; 100 minutes at 9.0 METs is near the top of the recommended range.

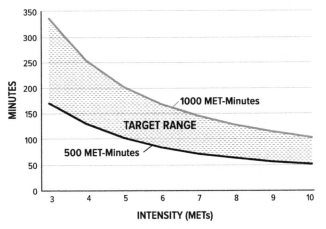

Figure 7: Recommended Weekly Physical Activity Range for U.S. Adults

Children ages six to seventeen need a recommended 60 minutes or more of moderate-to-vigorous-intensity aerobic physical activity (MVPA) per day.[4] That's an hour of exercise at a level of 3.0 METs or higher—basically walking briskly or running. At an average intensity of 4.0 METs, that means the minimum recommendation for children and adolescents is about twice that for adults:

420 minutes of movement x 4.0 METs = 1,680 MET-minutes per week.

The recommendation for children is not shown in figure 7 because intensity is so important for them that only a moderate-to-vigorous level provides any meaningful benefit. Since anything below 3.0 METs counts as 0, MET-minutes is not an ideal unit of measure for the recommendation. Nonetheless, the MET-minute equation is very helpful conceptually in understanding the importance of intensity when planning PA for youth.

Shortfalls in School PA

Now back to our California story. Imagine PA being led by a general classroom teacher there, or in any one of the 25 percent of schools nationwide that do not require PA teachers to have any "certification, licensure or endorsement by the state in physical activity."[5] This teacher quite possibly knows no more about PA than any of us do, beyond our shared cultural experience in elementary school gym class, with its repertoire of elimination, low-participation, and low-intensity games. And suppose that the teacher has decided to have the class play kickball.

At any moment, what is a given child most likely doing? The smart money is on standing, or possibly sitting on the floor. During a kickball game, only two or three people are in motion at a time (and usually not for long) while the rest wait for their turn to move. These kids are all getting effectively no PA.

And kickball is far from the only example. Dodgeball may actually be the worst offender because it combines a low overall dose of activity with a concentration of that dose in the children who are already the most skilled and fit. The kids who got hit in the back during the first five seconds watch as the last couple of athletes duke it out for 10 minutes or more, further honing their skills and fitness—thus making dodgeball the PA equivalent of the rich getting richer.

To encourage a higher dose of activity and help kids meet daily minimums, the CDC recommends that schools ensure that at least 50 percent of all students' activity time is spent moving at an MVPA intensity level. They call this threshold "one of the most critical outcome measures in determining the quality of a physical education [or activity] program."[6] However, a CATCH study concluded that only 21 percent of U.S. schools meet this minimum guideline.[7]

How to Increase Both Time and Intensity

Many schools have shown creativity in increasing physical activity by incorporating movement into classroom settings and providing it in short bursts during the school day. This certainly helps with the time side of the equation, and with the right activity selection, it can help with the intensity side, too.

The "activity break" at the end of Part II is an example of a brief, moderate-intensity activity that can be easily performed in a classroom. Another example, called "Zero In," incorporates math and is appropriate for kids aged eight to eleven. A student volunteer stands at the front of the class, facing the rest of the students as the teacher holds up a card with a problem behind her head so only her classmates can see it. (Let's say it's 210 divided by 3.) Then the teacher says, "Everyone help her find this number, which is between 0 and 500." If the volunteer guesses a number that is too high, the other students (and the volunteer) all do squats; if the volunteer guesses a number that is too low, everyone does jumping jacks, thereby helping her "zero in" on the correct answer of 70. Thus, in a few short minutes, it is possible for everyone to practice division and also get an activity break that stimulates and then settles their mind for further learning. A striking piece entitled "This Is Your Brain on Exercise" shows the dramatic increase in brain activity in someone who has just taken a walk compared to someone who has been sitting quietly.[8] Which kid do you want in your classroom?

Another way to increase PA across the student population is to limit exemptions that allow students to skip it in favor of a non-active extracurricular pursuit, to let them make up missed academic work, or as a form of discipline for an infringement. Schools need to adopt a culture in which physical activity is for everybody every day, rather than something that's discretionary, tailored for athletes, or a reward for good behavior.

By far the most powerful solution for increasing PA is

to ensure that anyone leading it, be they a classroom teacher or a specialist, receives regular and pertinent professional development with a focus on: 1) increasing students' MVPA; and 2) making PA varied and fun to help create lifelong positive attitudes about it. Just as improving your cooking involves both learning techniques and expanding your repertoire of recipes, improving PA requires that teachers learn specific class-management skills and also be exposed to new activities they can lead. Examples of techniques taught in PA training include keeping kids active during transitions, delivering concise instructions and signals, and including all students through offering non-elimination games and providing adaptations for those with special needs.

The importance of these basic practices in leading PA for kids reflects the fact that much valuable activity time can be wasted on class management. Too often, a teacher will start activity time like this, "OK, everyone, sit down and be quiet so I can explain today's activity." Kids have already been sitting quietly for hours when they finally get to the gym, and being sedentary is exactly what they're dying to get away from. So it is easy for their restlessness to translate into acting out, further prolonging the time allotted for delivering directions in an escalating cycle.

PA leaders can be taught to more effectively manage this transition time by making it active. For example, they can start class by having everyone "hit the track," walking or jogging around the perimeter of the gym while instructions are given. Teachers can also learn to give more concise signals and involve students in delivering them. For example, instead of clapping and imploring, "Everyone please be quiet now and listen," a teacher can say, "If you can hear me clap once," then clap once in unison with the kids, and then say slightly louder, "If you can hear me, clap twice," then clap twice in unison with the kids. This approach brings the class to attention with remarkable speed.

A third vital technique for leading PA to maximize MVPA is to ensure that all kids are included all of the time. This means making sure that the general population of kids—not just the athletes—are participating fully. It also extends to children with intellectual and physical disabilities whose needs are more complex. Practices for fostering full participation include adjustments such as changing "freeze tag" (which involves kids ceasing movement when tagged) to "jumping jack tag" (which has them stop running but still keeps them moving when tagged). Adaptations for special-needs kids may be more significant, like replacing jumping rope with simple hopping or even squatting.

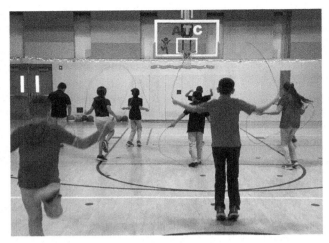

Making PA participatory, vigorous, and fun at Jefferson Elementary School, Edinburg, Texas! (Photograph by CATCH Global Foundation. Used with permission.)

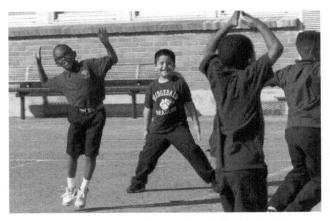

Students playing at Bridgedale Elementary School, Metairie, Louisiana (Photograph by CATCH Global Foundation. Used with permission.)

These PA management skills take time and practice to learn and perfect, and they are typically outside of the training and experience of a general classroom teacher.

That's a big part of the reason that three-quarters of U.S. schools deliver PA using certified specialists.[9] Although training can help academic teachers meet MVPA minimums, it cannot fully close the gap with specialists in this area. Nor can it arm generalists with an equal range of activities (for kids, variety is fun), or enable them to teach lifelong physical skills like locomotor movement, ball handling, and agility. Unfortunately, the facts that 25 percent of schools leave teaching physical activity entirely to general classroom teachers and that 41 percent of schools don't require any continuing education for physical educators, mean that kids in close to half of all U.S. schools are getting physical activity led by someone with no credentials or up-to-date training.[10]

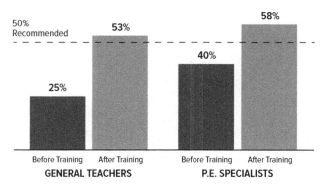

Figure 8: Portion of Structured Activity Time Children Spent in MVPA, Before and After Teacher Training[11]

How Higher PA Intensity Creates More Time

Figure 8 illustrates the cumulative impact that teacher specialization and training can make on kids' ability to attain the level of PA intensity required for good health.

Hiring credentialed teachers and training them regularly provides students with the most appropriate activities and has been found to increase kids' exercise intensity from an average of 40 percent MVPA to 58 percent MVPA.[12] That level of improvement offers the same aerobic benefit as lengthening an activity period from 30 minutes to 43 minutes, but without actually adding a single minute to the school schedule!

Let's stop thinking only about the first half of the minutes-*times*-intensity physical activity equation, which values effort without regard for results. We need to shift the debate from the number of PA minutes we can squeeze into a crowded school schedule to how to maximize the minutes we already have. Schools should ensure that the time allotted to PA produces moderate-to-vigorous physical activity for all kids, just as the time allotted to math is expected to produce moderate-to-vigorous multiplication activity for all kids.

Summary

The educational system can help students by shifting its focus from the amount of time devoted to physical activity to the amount of physical activity performed, which is the product of time and intensity. Simple, regular training can enable both general teachers and physical education specialists to provide more aerobic value, and thus more health and academic value, from the physical activity minutes already on school schedules.

Recommended Actions

Parents of school-age children: Ask your school how they train PA leaders and measure PA intensity to ensure that all kids are getting the minimum recommended aerobic activity dose.

Teachers: Seek opportunities to add activity breaks to the classroom and (in younger grades) to transition time.

Principals: Be resourceful in meeting or exceeding district guidelines, ensuring 24 hours of health education per year and 30 minutes of moderate-to-vigorous physical activity per day for every child. Use before-school time and minutes already allocated to PE, lunchroom, homeroom, and/or advisory group meetings. Encourage classroom teachers to add activity breaks, which can reinforce learning to their routine.

School boards, superintendents, and district administrators: Require letter-grade PE classes that include at least 30 minutes per day of moderate-to-vigorous intensity physical activity for every student. Ensure regular professional development for anyone leading physical activity.

Lawmakers and education policy makers: Fund health and physical activity with accountability for outcomes (such as activity levels) not process (such as minutes spent).

CASE STUDY

Teachers in Action—Sparkle Cheer at Del Valle High School, Del Valle, Texas

A cheer team comprising general- and special-education students delights students, parents, teachers, and community members while modeling inclusion and healthy fun.

The earth is flat as far as the eye can see around Del Valle High School in Central Texas, and trees are in short supply. With 78 percent of students eligible for FRL here, you might expect to find the type of social challenges that disproportionately affect low-income schools, such as teen pregnancy, gang affiliation, and fighting. But in the gym, something very unusual and progressive is going on.

Origin Story

It began in 2015, when the mother of a special-needs student asked Cheer Coach, Shana Green, whether it would be possible to get a uniform for her daughter, since she admired the athletes so much. Green recalls pausing for a moment and thinking, "Maybe we go further and actually put special-education kids on a team? I think we can do this!"

Coach Green first researched the idea and was pleased to identify a national organization, The Sparkle Effect, that supports varsity cheer teams who mentor special-needs students, including having them suit up in uniform for occasional appearances together. She says that although the organization was very encouraging, and inspired Del Valle High's program name, the program didn't meet the needs of Del Valle students.

A New Model

So Green went her own way and partnered with Structured Learning Teacher, Kelcey Williams, to create "Sparkle Cheer," an inclusive team comprising students in both of the school's learning programs: general (for students without disabilities) and structured (for students with intellectual and/or physical disabilities). The Sparkle team is separate from the varsity and JV cheer teams, which allows Sparkle to have daily practices and multiple performance opportunities. Sparkle routines are choreographed based on the needs and capabilities of its members. For example, a general-education student may do a tumbling pass followed by another general education student pushing a special education team member in a wheelchair through another pass.

Special education students are also included in stunts, which always include careful safety precautions. A common practice on cheer teams is to have a "big sister" or brother paired with a "little sister" or brother. This type of partnership works well for Sparkle. "Bigs" and "littles" pair up during warm-up each day and they shadow one another when developing and practicing new skills. Overall, Green and Williams found that the modifications needed to incorporate special-ed students into cheer routines were less extensive than they expected.

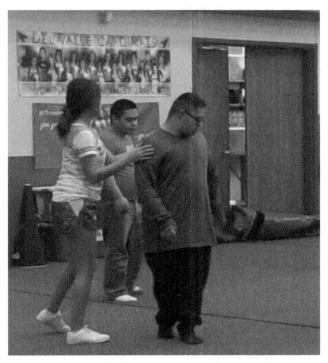

A general education student helps a special education student line up during Sparkle cheer practice (Photograph by CATCH Global Foundation. Used with permission.)

In establishing the Sparkle team, the teachers overcame several challenges. The first was convincing district administrators to allocate money and practice time for it. The organizers stressed that this team would foster inclusion of often-marginalized special-ed students as well as general-ed students whose skill was more in their ability to cooperate than in pure athleticism. The teachers quickly found that as a concept, "inclusion sells itself." And they were even able to secure a "varsity" designation for the Sparkle team—a big deal in terms of heightened status and sense of belonging for its members. The honor includes school-funded letter jackets and paid travel costs for one "away" competition per year.

The school could not cover the cost of uniforms, however, so Green negotiated discounts from the vendor so parents were able to cover the expense themselves. Green and Williams also identified discounted entry fees for special-athlete teams at competitions, reflecting the larger movement for inclusion in the sport of cheer. Finally, the teachers collaborated with Del Valle's athletic director and special-ed program administrators to secure disabled-accessible vehicles and to recruit volunteers to transport students to games.

Over its first four years, Sparkle has grown to about 30 members, divided about evenly between general- and special-education groups. Their accomplishments have added to the giant cheer trophy collection that rings its way around the school gymnasium. When Sparkle performs at football and basketball games, they enjoy rowdy standing ovations from the entire community.

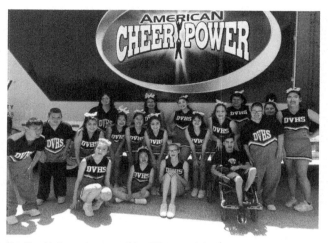

The Sparkle team at a competition (Photograph by Del Valle ISD. Used with permission.)

Impact

Williams says many of her special-needs students are nonverbal, but she can detect the impact of this activity on both their well-being and physical fitness. One team member frequently used a wheelchair through middle school but gained strength and confidence through Sparkle and was able to stop using it. Other students have actually made their first vocalizations while calling out cheers. Meanwhile, general-education team members have developed patience and practiced techniques for gently guiding their teammates and supporting their best efforts at participation. A number of them now aspire to careers in working with people with disabilities.

Former team captain, Vannessa Jaimes, captures her experience:

> My favorite moments in Sparkle were watching the team work hard every day at practice and seeing each and every one of them grow. I loved seeing how happy the team was to get into their cheer uniforms and have so many people cheer for them at games and competition. The school really responded to our team when we performed at pep rallies. Having the privilege to be on and captain the Sparkle team has made a huge impact on my life.

Principles of Effective Health Teaching

Del Valle High's Sparkle Cheer program models at least three elements of teaching health effectively in schools. First, it embodies the principle that physical activity programs need to be participatory and inclusive for all, not geared only to the best athletes. Second, it integrates youth empowerment and the development of social and emotional learning skills into health programming, in this case for both the general- and special-education students. And finally, Sparkle creates a shared celebration of health, uniting teachers, staff, students, and parents in a positive environment.

Certainly deserving of a big CHEER!

For more information about Del Valle High School's Sparkle Cheer program, or to make a donation to support it, please visit www.sparklecheer.org.

CHAPTER 9

CELEBRATING NUTRITION: INVOLVING EVERYONE IS FREE AND FUN

How to harness the collective power of the entire school community to teach health.

Just as chapter 7 applies mostly to older K–12 kids, this chapter applies mostly to younger ones. Providing strong nutrition education and a celebratory environment of health to elementary school children helps healthy behaviors persist into adolescence, and many of the techniques described here can be adapted for that age group.

As we have seen, practicing good health habits is a social and emotional behavior. For healthy habits to stick, teaching health needs to be participatory and it needs to be fun. A long-time CATCH saying captures this concept in a uniquely Texan way: "If it ain't fun, it don't get done!"

Principles of Nutrition Education for Children: GO-SLOW-WHOA

CATCH builds its nutrition education program on three key principles:

1. minimizing intake of foods and beverages with extensive processing and added salt and sugar
2. favoring plant-based foods such as whole grains, fruits, and vegetables
3. controlling portion size.

To help simplify these ideas and communicate them in a memorable way, CATCH uses the labels GO, SLOW, and WHOA to categorize foods by their relative nutritional value. (These terms were developed by nutritionists and health educators as part of the first version of CATCH, which was funded by the National Heart, Lung and Blood Institute, and their definitions have been updated several times as nutrition science has evolved.) Each category has a corresponding green, yellow, or red stoplight color. Kids embrace this system intuitively as early as Pre-K. After all, what child isn't fascinated with all things transportation?

GO foods are whole foods with limited processing, added salt, or added sugar (such as an apple); SLOW foods have been lightly processed or contain a few added ingredients (such as fruit canned in light syrup); WHOA foods have the most processing and added ingredients (such as ice cream). Kids can quickly learn to categorize foods accordingly, with the goal of eating more

GO foods than SLOW foods, and more SLOW foods than WHOA foods in a given day. Appropriate portion sizes are also emphasized. This holistic approach helps limit energy intake without counting calories and goes beyond imparting knowledge to reinforcing the social and behavioral dimensions of nutrition. Because it's about choices, not absolutes, this system reduces perfectionism about food selection (there are no NO foods) and avoids shaming kids about eating small amounts of less-nutritious foods on a limited basis. Since it is not a diet or rigid food list, the GO-SLOW-WHOA framework can be culturally adapted and modified to address food allergies.

Plant-based foods are increasingly recognized as critical to nutrition because they provide valuable nutrients such as antioxidants, which reduce cell damage, and immunity-boosting phytochemicals, which are essentially part of the plant's own immune system. In addition, plant-based foods are a good source of fiber, which helps to promote a healthy gut microbiome—all of the bacteria and other organisms that aid in digestion and other regulatory functions. Whole grains, fruits, and vegetables that are prepared without fat, salt, or processing are categorized as GO or SLOW foods, so the importance of plant-based foods is built into the GO-SLOW-WHOA classification system.

Developing Positive Attitudes about Nutrition

A great way to put these principles into action is to turn

the lunchroom into a nutrition education classroom (see case study on "Principal in Action" following chapter 3). Schools have worked hard over the past generation to make cafeteria food more nutritious, but it's not just about what's on the menu. It's about how healthy foods are *promoted*, as that drives not just what kids put into their mouths but also how they feel about it. Those attitudes and beliefs, in turn, affect the nutritional choices they make outside of school and in the future.

There are many ways to condition kids' attitudes about food, and all of them are essentially free. For example, research has demonstrated that fun and empowering names for healthy foods increase young children's willingness to taste, consume, and enjoy them.[1] Change carrots to "night-vision carrots" and rebrand broccoli as "bulging bicep broccoli." Adding labeling or putting up posters to communicate these concepts also helps animate blank school walls. Yet, according to the CDC, only 39 percent of schools "label healthful items with an appealing, age-appropriate name." Only 44 percent conduct taste tests with kids (in which everyone is invited to sample a small portion of an unusual food), and only 45 percent put up signage anywhere outside the cafeteria promoting healthy eating.[2]

What's even better is kid-created messaging. Have students make the signs and invent the food names so they develop a sense of ownership and reinforce health principles in their own minds. These basic principles of empowerment work in middle and high school too. Adolescents paint still lifes in art class anyway, so why not have a "healthy food" painting contest and display the winners in the cafeteria? At all ages, the best way to learn is to teach, and the best way to believe is to evangelize.

Another way to turn the lunch routine into fun and memorable health education is to have teachers and staff dress up as their favorite fruits and vegetables or walk around with a microphone and interview students about which healthy foods they're eating and why. And you can rename the lunchroom something playful using the school mascot, like the "Beagle Bistro." Kids also love special theme days, such as "Tasting Tuesday," when they taste samples of seasonal vegetables, or "Fruity Friday," when everyone wears a shirt or accessory in the color or their favorite fruit and gets to tell their classmates what that is. Finally, a school-based activity that kids particularly enjoy and that fosters positive attitudes about nutrition is creating a school garden. Children love the whole process, from preparing to planting to watering and especially, to harvesting the bounty. Tasting a vegetable that one has grown and picked is an entirely different experience from tasting one that has been fully prepared by someone else.

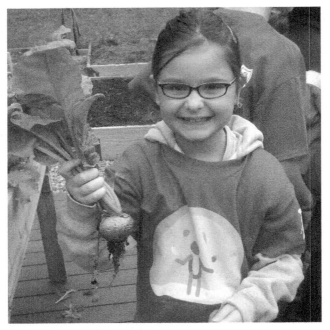

Can't "beet" the feeling of growing your own vegetables (Photograph by New Jersey YMCA State Alliance. Used with permission.)

Involve Cafeteria Staff

When you start thinking about ways to promote nutritious eating in school by making the cafeteria a fun place, you may realize that the oft-overlooked cafeteria workers are in fact some of the most important health educators of all. They know the kids' names and are in an excellent position to encourage healthy food choices. If we can't raise their wages, can we give them a status raise, some training, membership on the School Wellness Team, or other recognition and empowerment as part of the school's commitment to health?

The communication and coordination gap between health education and nutrition services is yawning. Less than half of schools involve nutrition services staff in any health education, and only 25 percent involve health educators in any nutrition services.[3] Think of the lost opportunities for joyful creativity, not to mention positive collaboration.

Gather Together

In developing strategies for creating a culture of health, principals, parents, and other school leaders should remember that health is social. So the most powerful way they can communicate its importance is to *show up* (another principle of SCT; see chapter 5). Principals can drop in on PE class once per term or better yet participate personally. Parents can join the School Wellness Team or ask regularly about its activities and progress. Fundraisers based on selling unhealthy fare like candy and cookies can be replaced with healthier, participatory alternatives such as dance-a-thons and seasonal fruit fairs in cooperation with local farmers. All of us can respond to appeals for our time and money with a short appearance and token pledge to demonstrate our commitment to healthy behavior in a way that is visible to kids and staff.

Another important way to combine health communication and celebration (and potentially, fundraising) is by holding school events for parents and community members. It's often hard to get parents involved, but many schools find that health is one of the best ways to hook them. Some schools hold a PE open house one evening per semester, when kids and parents can be active together. It is a magical experience for children to discover that the school is still there at night, to show off their independence and skills, and to experience the unbelievable hilarity of seeing the principal dressed as a banana.

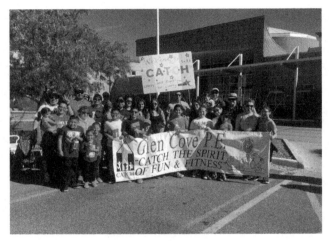

Parents and students at Glen Cove Elementary in El Paso, Texas show their Whole Community spirit of health (Photograph by Ysleta ISD. Used with permission.)

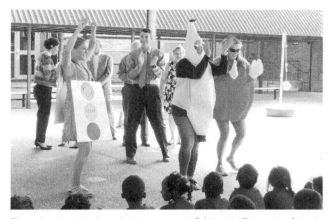

The author (center) at a celebratory event at Bridgedale Elementary School, Metairie, Louisiana (Photograph by CATCH Global Foundation. Used with permission.)

Further, events like this inoculate families with a dose of the health-behavior modeling and health-vocabulary building their kids receive at school, which they can then reinforce outside the classroom. And the emotional high of being active together strengthens community bonds long after the gym lights have been shut off.

Communication Is Part of Health

Make sure to capture the fun of these activities in short videos and share them across the school's social media channels. Since health behaviors are inherently social, connecting the community in this manner is not an add-on to teaching health; it is *part* of teaching health. As my teenage daughters remind me these days, if it's not happening on social media, it's basically not happening at all.

Once schools prioritize a culture of health and set a program in motion, they often find that kids quickly become the best health ambassadors of all. Health education is a great opportunity for youth empowerment because children readily adopt the language and norms of health. In a form of positive peer pressure, then they recruit their friends and parents into joining them in health-protective behaviors including regular exercise, nutritious eating, and tobacco and vaping avoidance. Observational learning does not require the role model to be older than the learner! Although pessimists may see health education as a constant uphill battle, the results are almost miraculous when we tap into children's natural desire to be and feel healthy.

Summary

School cafeterias should be part of nutrition education, and cafeteria staff part of teaching health. Effective health education isn't something one teacher does in one classroom. Creating a healthy school community requires including everyone in community-wide practices and celebrations, all of which can be achieved at little to no cost.

Recommended Actions

Parents of school-age children: Be generous in devoting time and money to school health-related activities and appeals, even if that is only one hour or one dollar. Support healthy fundraisers like activity challenges, not unhealthy ones like cookie sales.

Teachers: Initiate and participate in school health activities and be a health leader among faculty.

Principals: Elevate health educators and health education to first-class status through recognition and celebration of teacher, cafeteria staff, and student role models. Participate personally in the process of teaching and celebrating health.

School boards, superintendents, and district administrators: Develop staffing and accountability systems that ensure teaching health is a priority at every school. For example, require health to be included in school improvement plans, observe your school's culture of health in walk-throughs, and evaluate principals on measures such as students' health attitudes, beliefs, and MVPA.

CASE STUDY

Food Service in Action—Altus Public Schools, Altus, Oklahoma

*The food service team in a rural district leads
an all-hands effort to deliver meals to students
during COVID-19 school closures.*

The town of Altus sits in the southwest corner of Oklahoma and is rural, remote, and prone to extreme summer heat, reaching temperatures as high as 120 degrees. With flat topography, its every road runs as a north-south or east-west gridline. After hitting a high of 23,302 residents in 1970, Altus' population has declined by 20 percent over the past five decades. And, as of the 2010 census, 23 percent of Altus' children under 18 lived below the federal poverty line. These demographics paint Altus as a textbook example of the economic and social hardships that have hit rural America over the past 50 years. But the community boasts a tough, proud cohesion and a sense of discipline inspired, perhaps, by the nearby Air Force base.

On the afternoon of March 12, 2020, Altus Public Schools' Superintendent, Roe Worbes, came into the office of the district's Director of Child Nutrition, Sabina Garrett. He informed her that the next day, its schools would be closing due to the coronavirus outbreak, with no reopening date in sight. "What can we do to keep our 3,500 kids fed?" he asked. Garrett worked into the night drafting a plan—and Operation Bulldog Thunder was born.

Operation Bulldog Thunder

This program offered 10 free meals per week (breakfast and lunch, Monday through Friday) for 10 weeks to all residents of Altus ages 18 and under, plus disabled kids up to age 21. After its rollout on March 23, it provided a total of 129,794 meals to students—an average of 2,600 each weekday.

All the food was prepared in the kitchen of Altus High School (home of the Bulldogs), by eight to ten district staff cooks working full time in eight-day shifts starting at 6:00 each morning. Volunteers bagged the food for delivery via six district school buses, which brought it to 21 stops throughout the city; cars served outlying areas. When buses arrived with food, they were often met by lines of hungry children stretching for blocks.

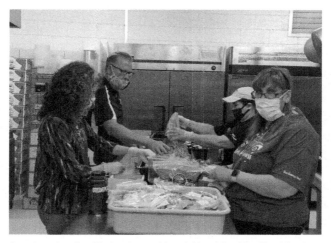

Superintendent Roe Worbes (second from left) and the Altus Food Service team pack vegetables for students during Operation Bulldog Thunder. Health is a team sport! (See chapters 6 and 9.) (Photograph by Altus Public Schools. Used with permission.)

Garrett describes how, as the planning started, she quickly realized that this effort was analogous to a military deployment (thus requiring an appropriate-sounding name). So she called on her experience from years in the service, organizing the work into four categories: funding, food supply, labor, and communications. Before the details were final, Superintendent Worbes asked her to start making the arrangements for buying and cooking the food; he would ensure that the school district funded the program.

It did. At first, the district tapped funds from the USDA's Seamless Summer Option, an emergency food program it had used previously during a period of teacher strikes. To obtain more reimbursement and flexibility in menu planning, it quickly switched to another USDA program, Summer Food Service, which has ended up covering most of the cost of the operation. In order to provide extra whole grains and fresh fruits and vegetables in their meals, Altus Public Schools also tapped the USDA's Commodity Supplemental Food Program and its Fresh Fruit and Vegetable Program, along with accepting contributions from the community. In all, they received more than $21,000 in funding, including $10,000 in a single check—which brought Garrett to tears.

Even with money to buy the food, obtaining it was not easy. District vendors faced supply-chain disruptions and overwhelming demand as people fearfully stockpiled groceries. Garrett was on the phone with suppliers at all hours to ensure deliveries to run the program and worked especially hard to secure fresh produce.

People power turned out to be less of an issue. Oklahoma's Governor, Kevin Stitt, had generously arranged for all school district personnel in the state to be paid throughout the period of school closures. However, no one was required to report to work, so Operation Bulldog Thunder essentially depended on volunteerism for both the skilled labor of cooking and the unskilled labor of packaging and clean-up. Fortunately, a large number of people pulled together and answered the call. In fact, so many district teachers and staff wanted to help that Garrett assigned them to shifts first, before accepting parent and other community member volunteers. Maintaining proper nutrition and offering a fun variety of foods that kids enjoyed often meant extra work bagging individual items, but the team did not flinch. One day they even served sloppy joes, which were a giant hit with both kids and parents!

The final dimension of coordinating this project was publicizing it, an especially challenging task considering the project had to go from idea to launch in 12 days. Garrett worked with the district's communications office to publish information about the program and maps of delivery sites on the district's website, and later to create YouTube videos and Facebook posts. But since many student families do not have reliable internet access, the district also needed to spread the word through traditional media. Thankfully, they were able to secure TV coverage for the program on local ABC News affiliate KSWO.

After Operation Bulldog Thunder concluded at the end of May, local children began receiving meals through a collaboration Garrett arranged with Meals-to-You, a nationwide food delivery-by-mail program run by the USDA and Baylor University in Waco, Texas. As of this writing, it will run through August 15, 2020, and district personnel are working to figure out how to continue providing food if schools are not reopened in August.

Building on Previous Work

To understand the conditions that made Operation Bulldog Thunder so successful, so quickly requires looking back at the work Garrett and Altus's Food Service

Department were doing *before* the COVID-19 crisis hit. Altus already had important physical infrastructure and know-how, running two programs to increase students' access to healthy foods.

First, while many U.S. school districts offer free breakfast in the cafeteria to eligible students, Altus was part of a much smaller group that offered it in the classroom prior to the commencement of the school day. This format requires extra labor (to distribute food and clean up classrooms) but has the advantage of reaching more kids by serving them where they already are and eliminating the effort of going to the cafeteria. Thanks to this program, the district already had equipment such as carts and coolers, which proved invaluable for moving food in Operation Bulldog Thunder. It also owned three hydroponic lettuce-growing machines to help provide salads, bought with an earlier grant and used at full capacity during the operation.

Second, for the past eight years, Altus had run a summer food program that served meals to about 225 students per day. Although it required kids to come to school to pick up the meals, plans were already in place to add a delivery option in 2020. The logistics behind this smaller-scale program proved to be crucial in mounting the emergency operation by establishing routines for food preparation during school closures.

More broadly, Altus's Food Services team has long gone far beyond the minimum of providing food to take a leadership role in promoting health. In addition to her "day job" leading Food Services, Garrett heads the district's wellness committee. In this role, she coordinates and advises on functions, such as classroom health education, physical education, and the overall school wellness environment—signage, parent communications, and health-related events. In other words, Garrett orchestrates the district's entire Whole Child health model, using the Oklahoma State Department of Health's Certified Healthy Oklahoma School Program as a guide.

Around the country, it is uncommon for a school's food service department (variously called "cafeteria management," "child nutrition services," etc.) to actively participate in wider health initiatives at that school. The fact that food service is considered part of teaching health and wellness at Altus Public Schools is commendable. That food service *leads* the overall effort is truly remarkable, or as Garrett says simply, "It's huge!"

Altus Public Schools uses the CATCH program as a foundation for its Whole Child wellness work. Garrett's Food Services group oversees the following initiatives, all of which are led by existing teachers and staff using existing resources:

- ensuring that health topics (many of which are included in state standards) are actually taught in the classroom
- providing physical education activities that reinforce nutrition concepts

- encouraging creation and posting of signs depicting the GO-SLOW-WHOA food classification system in cafeterias and classrooms
- requiring each school to designate a CATCH champion and wellness team that reports quarterly to Garrett on their activities and progress.

Altus has also embraced the concept that food service staff are frontline health educators. Each summer, the district pays a group of their child nutrition professionals to attend Oklahoma State University's Cooking for Kids Skill Development Training. The Cooking for Kids program is funded by the Oklahoma State Department of Education Child Nutrition and provides free, chef-led culinary training to school districts in Oklahoma. Altus's participation also makes the district eligible to have a Cooking for Kids chef come to its schools and work with students, supplementing the formal nutrition education provided in classrooms and during physical education. Among other things, the chef conducts cooking demonstrations and holds sessions focused on tasting unusual fruits and vegetables and learning where and how they are grown.

The Cooking for Kids program has also helped improve recipes and menus offered at the schools and helped the staff set up an initiative to allow Pre-K and kindergarten children to get a pre-boxed entrée salad for lunch instead of a hot meal when they want to. About one hundred kids choose this option each day, helping them to consume more vegetables without having to piece together their own salad from a salad bar—a big barrier for young children.

Through these initiatives, Garrett—like all good leaders—has created a culture of health within the district and nurtured participation from her own team, her supervisor, teachers, and staff in other departments, and parents. When she fought to get "hydration stations" (basically vertical water fountains to refill water bottles) in every school, teachers told her how much they enjoyed using them. When she launched the pre-boxed salad option, parents "lit up" Facebook with appreciation. When she came to her superintendent with ideas, she showed she could find government and community programs and dollars to fund them.

The substantial work the Food Services team has done to make health a priority at Altus Public Schools has delivered excellent health education during usual times and exceptional heroism during unusual times.

CHAPTER 10

CATCH: DOING GOOD, SCALING GREAT

CATCH, one of the largest school health programs in the world, has scaled up to reach 3 million kids per year through a unique collaboration among scientists, philanthropists, grassroots school and community leaders, and a nonprofit organization dedicated to its expansion.

Coordinated Approach To Child Health (CATCH) is one of the largest and most scientifically rigorous Whole Child health and wellness programs in the world—as well as my employer and the basis for much of the material in this book. As I mentioned in chapter 1, this book exists to promote a big idea about the value of teaching health in schools, not CATCH specifically, so I will only include a short summary here and refer you to CATCH. org for more details. Then I will focus on the four enduring structural principles behind CATCH's success and provide an example of how this structure uniquely enabled it to mount a rapid response to the youth vaping epidemic over the past four years.

CATCH Snapshot

As of 2020, CATCH provides evidence-based Whole Child health programming to 15,000 educational sites worldwide (mostly in the U.S.), reaching 3 million Pre-K–12 youth annually and untold tens of millions cumulatively. CATCH offers curricula, materials, and training for: PE and PA; nutrition education; youth vaping prevention (CATCH My Breath, see below); integration with SEL and mental health programs; and Whole Child health policy, systems, and environment (PSE). Through evidence in more than 120 peer-reviewed scientific paper reviews and countless project evaluations, CATCH has demonstrated effectiveness in achieving three main behavioral outcomes among youth: increasing MVPA, increasing healthy food choices, and decreasing tobacco and vaping initiation.[1,2]

CATCH Principle No. 1: A Focus on Prevention

CATCH was created and tested through a pioneering 1988 grant from the NIH's National Heart, Lung, and Blood Institute (NHLBI) to a group of five research institutions: New England Research Institute, Tulane University School of Public Health and Tropical Medicine, University of California San Diego, University of Minnesota, and The University of Texas. The program began with physical activity and nutrition education modules and expanded over time to add training and materials for tobacco prevention and support of a Whole Child wellness environment.

Over 30 years, CATCH has received funding targeted to addressing youth cardiovascular health, diabetes, obesity, cancer, and most recently, vaping. The fact that a single program promoting MVPA, nutritious food choices, and tobacco avoidance would be used for prevention of so many different disease endpoints testifies to the long-term, multipurpose impact of these foundational health behaviors. Since CATCH addresses the "upstream" behavioral causes of noncommunicable disease rather than the symptoms, it has been able to weather the sometimes-faddish government and philanthropic funding cycles rushing to address the "downstream" problem of the moment.

CATCH Principle No. 2: An Ongoing Cycle of Scientific Development and Real-World Feedback

Thanks to CATCH's unusual, ongoing relationship with one of its five parent research institutions (The University of Texas, specifically UTHealth School of Public Health and MD Anderson Cancer Center), science is part of our daily routine. Often, health education programs with a university pedigree (to say nothing of those without one) have a linear lifecycle, with the science done first and distribution afterwards. On the other hand, CATCH curricula, programs, and trainings are developed, tested, and updated through an ongoing cycle incorporating ever-evolving theory, measurement, and community feedback.

Scientific validity is an indispensable part of the success of any health education program, and because health and human behavior are complicated, such a program must be built on more than something someone made up in a conference room that seems likely to work. Evaluating the results of a health education program is a scientific process, too. It needs to be done impartially and the findings need to be replicated before something can confidently be labeled "evidence based." Unfortunately, many youth health programs—including some well-funded ones—offer little to no evidence of their actual health impact and may not even try to measure it.

Those programs that do get positive results may rely on a solitary one-and-done study to back them up. Other programs accumulate evidence over many years but aren't able to raise ongoing funding for updates. All in all, communities are often left with an unpleasant choice between a health education program that's current and one that's proven. CATCH is both.

CATCH Principle No. 3: A Nonprofit "Translational" Organization Dedicated to Community Empowerment and Sustainability

Unfortunately, research institutions that are qualified to create and evaluate youth health education programs are rarely set up to perform the ongoing work of helping communities to implement and sustain these programs. The converse is also true. Community-based organizations specializing in program support usually cannot do highly scientific program design and testing. As a consequence, many health education programs either languish on a university shelf or are contrived by well-meaning community organizations lacking scientific credibility.

So, in 2014, I participated in founding CATCH Global Foundation, an organization designed for "translational science:" bridging the gap between research and practice. Our dissemination experts package and market proven programs for large-scale use, provide consulting and technical assistance to communities wishing to implement them, and then return feedback from the real world to our university and philanthropic partners to support ongoing improvements and investments.

The CATCH model empowers communities by helping them to build the capacity to teach health themselves rather than doing it for them. Using principles of SCT and DOI (see chapter 5), we identify and train thought leaders within a community to serve as inspiring role models, communicating with their neighbors, peers, and students on familiar territory and in familiar terms. Decades ahead of the corporate trend of identifying "brand advocates" for word-of-mouth marketing, CATCH has always made amplifying community voices our primary communications strategy. We also cultivate grassroots ownership in other ways, such as by encouraging communities to add their own local flavor to CATCH. For example, one school in New Orleans created a Mardi Gras-themed bulletin board labeled "Throw Me Something Healthy!" Sometimes schools devise their own CATCH logo, acronym, or T-shirt designs in a joyous celebration of their own spirit of health. Surely imitation is the best form of dissemination!

And it is CATCH community leaders—not CATCH Global Foundation staffers—who institutionalize and sustain health education at the schools using our programs. Often, CATCH programs last through several generations of management turnover. When I ask, "How long has your school been using CATCH?" I am always flattered to hear, "I don't know, it was here when I arrived." This community ownership extends beyond implementation of CATCH to the science behind it. Many communities' projects include a university research partner and/or a formal evaluation methodology, which can fuel the scientific cycle described in Principle No. 2 independent of the CATCH team. It is not uncommon for CATCH to learn of new scientific research on its program only when a paper appears in a journal or is presented at a conference.

CATCH Principle No. 4: Finding the Sweet Spot

Ideally, mission-driven work happens at the intersection of what works scientifically, what communities want, and what gets funded. (See figure 9.) However, the last criterion—having enough money—often far outweighs the others in importance, sometimes to the point of superseding them. This dynamic has two damaging implications, which CATCH has sought to address.

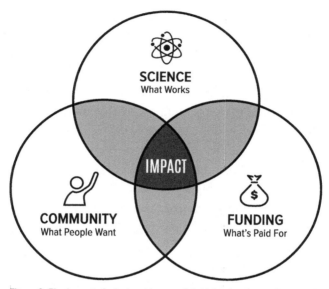

Figure 9: The impact of mission-driven work is highest at the confluence of science, community demand, and funding

First, community projects are sometimes funded before demand is properly established and end up chasing sparse interest, leading to disappointing participation and a lack of sustainability once the funding is gone. This risk is not news to many philanthropists, who increasingly look for clear evidence of community support before proceeding with a grant. Some value this consideration to the exclusion of all else. I have had funders (big ones!) tell me that their *only* criterion is community demand, even if the intervention that people say they want has no scientific merit. CATCH only offers programs that have been proven effective and never accepts gifts or grants for projects without demand from the community partner documented in advance. In establishing that interest, CATCH employs DOI, ensuring that there are thought leaders ready to undertake change and willing to evangelize that change to others.

The second and more concerning effect of the primacy of funding is that potentially powerful and necessary work may not get done in a timely manner. The process of cultivating and confirming community demand is long, and adding another long process of fundraising after that risks missing windows of opportunity. CATCH has addressed this timing problem by maintaining larger financial reserves than most nonprofits of its size, allowing it the flexibility to seed its own investments as soon as a promising opportunity arises. This practice also allows CATCH to groom and vet projects through their pilot phases before bringing them to outside funders, who are typically more conservative and like to see momentum and signs of success before investing. So, while CATCH applies for fewer grants than some similar organizations, its batting average is extraordinarily high.

CATCH My Breath: A Rapid Response to the Youth Vaping Epidemic

The four principles discussed above have figured prominently in CATCH's response over the past five years to the youth vaping epidemic. In 2014, years before anyone even used the word "epidemic" to describe the vaping problem, the Surgeon General's office commissioned UTHealth as the scientific editors of a report on youth vaping. Seeing both the threat and huge gaps in public awareness, UTHealth approached CATCH about collaborating on a school-based prevention program (see principle No. 2). Of course, there was no funding available to develop this idea, but after validating demand from nearby schools in Austin and health department partners, CATCH and UTHealth worked together off-hours to draft a curriculum (see principle No. 4).

In-school testing of CATCH My Breath began in late 2015, so by the time CATCH approached St. David's Foundation for a grant in mid-2016, it was able to show them early results and demonstrate community support from pilot schools. And although they had never funded CATCH before, St. David's knew of its reputation in other areas of K–12 health education (see principle Nos. 1 and 4).

Their grant enabled ongoing cycles of program refinement in collaboration with scientists and teachers, along with an evaluation comparing two sets of schools during the 2016–2017 school year. The results of the evaluation, which were published in a peer-reviewed journal, revealed a 46 percent decline in the number of seventh graders who had started vaping in schools that taught CATCH My Breath compared with seventh graders in schools who did not.[3] This finding made CATCH My Breath the first peer-reviewed, evidence-based youth vaping prevention program. It was then ready for prime time, and in the summer of 2017, CATCH won a generous grant from CVS Health to distribute the program nationwide (see principle No. 3).

Reach and Results

The rest, as they say, is history. During the 2017–2018 school year, CATCH My Breath reached approximately 50,000 youth in 200 schools nationwide; in 2018–2019, it grew to reach 350,000 youth in 1,100 schools; and in 2019–2020, it served over 1 million kids in 3,000 schools. The program is officially approved for use in five of the seven largest school districts in the country (Broward, Chicago, Houston, Miami-Dade, and New York City) and several other mega-districts including Dallas, Philadelphia, and Memphis. And it is now being offered throughout California in partnership with the California Department of Education. This steep growth would never have been possible without a collaborative effort between scientists, distribution experts, communities, and philanthropists, along with disciplined adherence to the CATCH principles and DOI.

So, good news: CATCH My Breath works, and communities like it! In addition to the peer-reviewed study mentioned above, CATCH's surveys of students who have completed the program have shown significant increases in their knowledge about e-cigarettes' health effects as well as positive changes in their beliefs, attitudes, and sense of empowerment:[4]

- 79 percent say they are less likely to vape because of the program.
- 81 percent say they are confident using a refusal skill learned in the program.
- 82 percent think *all* middle and high schoolers should go through CATCH My Breath.

That final point speaks volumes. If youth empowerment drives health behavior, and youth say they want to learn more about health, isn't that a good reason for schools to teach health?

PART IV

WHEN?

GOING BIG—BOLD IDEAS FOR THE FUTURE

CHAPTER 11

———

"WHEN AM I GOING TO USE THIS?"

Big-picture ideas for prioritizing
teaching health in K–12 schools.

The silver lining of our fragmented K–12 structure is that while no one holds all the power to make health a core priority, anyone who believes in an educational system focused on the development of healthy "Whole Children" can do something to move us in that direction. Educators are endlessly resourceful, and many have found ways to deploy the best practices we've discussed to fit a dose of health education into existing time and money budgets without sacrificing anything else. As we've discussed, some schools dedicate time from homeroom or advisory meetings to teaching health; some integrate health topics into science, language, or math curricula; and some use before-school, after-school, and lunch hours.

As this book has shown, many schools can still go a lot

further with teaching health for free—and that's a good immediate next step. But at some point, if we want to make big progress in teaching children about health, we will need to make some changes and invest more in providing it. Assuming no overall increases in time or money for education are forthcoming, to teach more health we will have to cut something else. How might we think about deciding what that would be?

Zero-Based Budgeting

The for-profit sector has developed a model that merits consideration: zero-based budgeting. Instead of allocating resources based on incremental up or down changes from the previous period, this technique has each demand fight for its place starting from scratch at the beginning of each planning cycle. Applying this concept literally is no doubt a waste of time when it comes to the K–12 curriculum, since we know kids need to learn 2+2 and the meaning of "courage." But a zero-based budgeting mindset has helped many organizations overcome the inertia of the past, challenge unseen and unspoken assumptions, and more quickly adapt their allocation of time and money to the demands of the present.

If we applied a zero-based approach to budgeting time in the school day, we would start by considering that each year, the average elementary school student spends:[1]

- 421 hours on English/Language Arts (ELA)
- 202 hours on math

- 83 hours on science
- 83 hours on history/social studies
- 41 hours on health (7 hours in classroom + 34 hours on physical education)[2]

In a zero-based budgeting conversation, we would ask questions such as "Is ELA 10 times more important than health? What would happen if we cut ELA by 10 percent, saving 42 hours per year, and then used them to double teaching time devoted to health? Is history twice as important as health? Can devoting more time to health make time spent learning ELA, math, science, and history more productive in the first place?"

The next level of detail would involve looking at specific topics that take up that school time and comparing their value: "Are the causes of World War I something everyone needs to know to be successful in life? Is how to prove right-triangle symmetry? Is how to resist peer and media pressure to use alcohol and tobacco?" Of course, all of these topics are important and school is for teaching abstract concepts as well as practical skills. But maybe it's time to drop just a few hours from ELA, or history, or geometry, so we can make time for our schools to teach the importance of nutrition also?

Such a suggestion would be shocking to many people, who might say: If our schools don't teach kids these subjects, who will—parents? Will our failure to teach these topics to everyone exacerbate social inequalities? And that's exactly the point. Since we can't assume that our nation's youth will get the ELA, math, and history education they need without learning it in school, how can we assume they will get the health education they need without learning it in school? Not giving everyone an adequate dose of health education may be exacerbating social inequalities just as much, or more.

If we are ever going to make health education a priority, we are going to need to shift the burden of proof from whether we can afford to take a minute from, say, history for health to whether we can afford to take a minute from health for history.

College-Admissions Departments

Since health drives academic success (see chapter 3), it would seem reasonable that college-admissions departments might perceive the value of knowing about the health knowledge, attitudes, and behaviors of their applicants. Such efforts would need to be approached with caution so as not to discriminate based on health status, which is different from health behavior. For example, admissions officers could seek evidence of applicants' practice of healthy behaviors (and avoidance of unhealthy ones) through interviews, recommendations, and choice of extracurricular activities. They could include a supplemental essay topic gauging applicants' health attitudes and behaviors, as well as their social and emotional skills, by asking about health routines or for examples of the applicant's use of SEL skills like self-management, social awareness, and responsible decision-making. Colleges could also use their influence on the K–12 standardized testing regime to encourage the College Board to assess health knowledge by adapting existing tests and creating new subject-specific ones.

Finally, many colleges already offer an orientation to incoming freshmen on health behaviors, such as sleep hygiene and stress management, because physical and mental health play such a crucial role in student performance. If understanding these issues is indeed important, why not move it a step earlier in the process and make health proficiency part of what students need to demonstrate to gain admission?

Beginning with the End in Mind

At some point, every parent and teacher has heard a schoolchild who was exasperated by a long day, a confusing concept, or an avalanche of facts pose the age-old question, "When am I going to use this?" We don't always have a great answer when it comes to certain obscure knowledge, but we have lots of ammo ready for the child who asks, "When am I going to use health?" if one ever does.

What would happen if we modeled the ideal of youth empowerment by asking that same question to help us decide what to cut to make more time for health?

Sooner or later, we all learn that the best way to look good and to feel good—and the common denominator in doctors' advice for managing most ailments and conditions—is to focus on "diet, exercise, and tobacco avoidance." From that point on, we use our health education literally every day. Can every topic in the K–12 curriculum make that claim?

If we are serious about ensuring that all kids have the right educational start to enable future success in life, when are we going to start teaching health as if each child's life depends on it? Because it does.

APPENDIX

SUMMARY OF RECOMMENDED ACTIONS BY ACTOR

Parents of School-Age Children

(Chapter 3) Band together to advocate for health education to your school principal. Cite the connections between health and learning and the term "Whole Child," especially if it is part of your district or school's mission or strategic plan.

(Chapter 5) In addition to discussing health facts, rehearse attitudes and social skills related to health with your children. Consider the health behaviors you are modeling at home.

(Chapter 6) Ask your school and district how they train and support teaching health, whether by general teachers or specialists.

(Chapter 7) Inform yourself about vaping basics and ask your school how they are addressing the epidemic.

(Chapter 8) Ask your school how they train PA leaders and measure PA intensity to ensure that all kids are getting the minimum recommended aerobic activity dose.

(Chapter 9) Be generous in devoting time and money to school health-related activities and appeals, even if that is only one hour or one dollar. Support healthy fundraisers like activity challenges, not unhealthy ones like cookie sales.

Teachers

(Chapter 3) Teach health with the passion, personal commitment, and student accountability that you put into other subjects.

(Chapter 6) Catch kids being healthy (i.e., practicing healthy behaviors and using health skills) and provide specific praise and positive reinforcement. Model healthy behavior, especially when you know students are watching.

(Chapter 7) Inform yourself about vaping basics and ask your school how they are addressing the epidemic.

(Chapter 8) Seek opportunities to add activity breaks to the classroom and (in younger grades) to transition time.

(Chapter 9) Initiate and participate in school health activities and be a health leader among faculty.

Principals

(Chapter 3) Understand and consider the mounting evidence that health impacts academic success.

(Chapter 5) Provide regular training and professional development for teachers on how to deliver effective health education that includes skill-building and social and emotional learning. Be systematic in identifying and empowering thought leaders.

(Chapter 6) Support the school health environment by making it a personal priority. Devote the same amount of time and attention to attending, observing, and evaluating School Wellness Team meetings, PE classes, and other health-related events and instruction that you give to reading and biology.

(Chapter 7) Provide youth vaping-prevention education proactively, rather than as a disciplinary response. Host a required informational session for staff and an optional one for parents.

(Chapter 8) Be resourceful in meeting or exceeding district guidelines, ensuring 24 hours of health education per year and 30 minutes of moderate-to-vigorous physical activity per day for every child. Use before-school time and minutes already allocated to PE, lunchroom, homeroom, and/or advisory group meetings. Encourage classroom teachers to add activity breaks, which can reinforce learning to their routine.

(Chapter 9) Elevate health educators and health education to first-class status through recognition and celebration of teacher, cafeteria staff, and student role models. Participate personally in the process of teaching and celebrating health.

School Boards, Superintendents, and District Administrators

(Chapter 3) Require the teaching of health in all K–12 schools, especially physical education and nutrition education, and especially in elementary schools.

(Chapter 5) Provide regular training and professional development for teachers on how to deliver effective health education that includes skill-building and social and emotional learning. Be systematic in identifying and empowering thought leaders.

(Chapter 6) "Put health on the test" by requiring and letter-grading 40 minutes per week of health education for every student (24 hours per school year).

(Chapter 7) Require evidence-based vaping prevention education for all students in grades five through twelve. (Although some experts advocate starting even sooner, others claim that can backfire by kindling curiosity.)

View the vaping epidemic as a symptom of a chronic lack of health education in schools, not an isolated problem to be overcome and forgotten.

(Chapter 8) Require and letter-grade PE classes that include at least 30 minutes per day of moderate-to-vigorous intensity physical activity for every student. Ensure regular professional development for anyone leading physical activity.

(Chapter 9) Develop staffing and accountability systems that ensure teaching health is a priority at every school. For example, require health to be included in school improvement plans, observe your school's culture of health in walk-throughs, and evaluate principals on measures such as students' health attitudes, beliefs, and MVPA.

Lawmakers and Education Policy Makers

(Chapter 3) Devise policies and incentives that drive schools to actively own, not just allow, health education.

(Chapter 5) Codify the definition of "health education" as addressing both knowledge and behavior acquisition.

(Chapter 6) Add or update health education competencies in state learning standards. Put accountability behind them by adding health as a subject in state standardized tests across the K–12 spectrum and measuring performance.

(Chapter 8) Fund health and physical activity with accountability for outcomes (such as activity levels) not process (such as minutes spent).

GLOSSARY

adverse childhood experiences (ACEs): According to the U.S. Department of Health and Human Services, these are traumatic events occurring before age 18. They include all types of abuse and neglect as well as parental mental illness, substance use, divorce, incarceration, and domestic violence.

Centers for Disease Control and Prevention (CDC): A U.S. federal agency that is part of the Department of Health and Human Services and is the nation's leading public health authority.

Diffusion of Innovations Theory (DOI): Pioneered by communications specialist and sociologist, Everett Rogers, this model explains the process by which new ideas and technologies spread.

Food and Drug Administration (FDA): A U.S. federal agency that is part of the Department of Health and Human Services and regulates tobacco products, among many other activities.

free or reduced-price lunch assistance (FRL): A U.S. federal government-supported program providing school meal subsidies for low-income students. Eligibility for FRL is often reported by school districts as a measure of "economic disadvantage."

Healthy Life Expectancy (HALE): A measure of life expectancy adjusted for health status, with years of life lived with disease or disability discounted based on the severity of that disease or disability.

health education: For specialists, this term usually means traditional in-classroom instruction only. For the broader audience of this book, I use this term (and the phrase "teaching health") more generally to encompass all forms of K–12 school-based instruction designed to teach health, including classroom learning, physical activity, physical education, and environmental support.

moderate-to-vigorous physical activity (MVPA): Physical activity performed at an intensity level of 3.0 METs or higher (see chapter 8 for a detailed explanation of METs).

physical activity (PA): Movement-focused time led by schoolteachers.

physical education (PE): Movement and physical skill-building time led by schoolteachers holding specific credentials in the subject.

Social Cognitive Theory (SCT): Developed by psychologist, Albert Bandura, a theory that human behavior is learned through reciprocal interaction among personal, social, and environmental factors.

social and emotional learning (SEL): As defined by The Collaborative for Academic, Social, and Emotional Learning (CASEL), the process through which children and adults understand and manage emotions, set and achieve positive goals, feel and show empathy for others, establish and maintain positive relationships, and make responsible decisions.

Whole Child: According to the Association for Supervision and Curriculum Development, an approach to education defined by policies, practices, and relationships that ensure each child, in each school, in each community, is healthy, safe, engaged, supported, and challenged. The phrases "Whole Child health" and "Whole Child wellness" are used synonymously.

ACKNOWLEDGMENTS

I am greatly indebted to many colleagues, friends, and loving family members for their advice and encouragement as I climbed this mountain of work.

First and most of all, thank you Kerry, Kate, and Judith for your honest and kind support, both silent and spoken.

Second, thank you to all of my CATCH teammates and community partners. You are the inspiration for this book!

And finally, thank you to the many other readers who saw me through 12 drafts over 2½ years. I received particularly helpful feedback from: Brooks Ballard, Kate Bellin, David Bocian, Rachelle Chiang, David Ginsburg, Shelby Goodrum, Leslie Hamilton, Denise Herrera, Chris Horan, Steve Kelder, Erin Maughan, Mark Peevy, the team at Scribe Publishing and, of course, my tireless editor, Miranda Spencer.

My profound appreciation to one and all!

ABOUT THE AUTHOR

DUNCAN VAN DUSEN is the Founder and CEO of CATCH Global Foundation, whose evidence-based "Whole Child" health programs reach over 15,000 schools and more than 3 million children annually. He has consulted with hundreds of schools on creating a culture of wellness, and speaks regularly on health behavior theory, health education, and the youth vaping epidemic.

Van Dusen completed his undergraduate education at Princeton University and earned his MPH from the University of Texas School of Public Health. He has authored peer-reviewed scientific papers in *Public Health Reports* and *Journal of School Health*. He enjoys spending time outdoors with his family and empowering his own daughters to exercise, avoid tobacco, and eat their vegetables.

NOTES & SOURCES FOR FURTHER READING

Chapter 1

1   "Healthy Life Expectancy (HALE) Data by Country," World Health Organization, https://apps.who.int/gho/data/node.main.HALE?lang=en.

2   "Developed Countries List 2020," World Population Review, https://worldpopulationreview.com/countries/developed-countries/ (using countries with an HDI of 0.85 or higher).

Chapter 2

1   Maya Riser-Kositsky, "Education Statistics: Facts About American Schools," *Education Week*, January 3, 2019, https://www.edweek.org/ew/issues/education-statistics/index.html.

2   Beth Resnick, et al., "An Examination of the Growing US Undergraduate Public Health Movement," *Public Health Reviews* 38, no. 4 (2017), https://publichealthreviews.biomedcentral.com/articles/10.1186/s40985-016-0048-x.

3   "Public Health Undergraduate Degree Options," University of Texas at Austin School of Human Ecology, https://he.utexas.edu/ph/undergraduate-degree.

4   Dan Kopf, "The 2008 Financial Crisis Completely Changed What Majors Students Choose," *Quartz*, August 29, 2018, https://qz.com/1370922/the-2008-financial-crisis-completely-changed-what-majors-students-choose/.

Case Study: Lawmakers in Action—New York City Department of Education

1   "DOE Data at a Glance," New York City Department of Education, https://www.schools.nyc.gov/about-us/reports/doe-data-at-a-glance.

2   Data from Niche, https://www.niche.com/k12.

3   Beth Fertig, "Mayor's Budget Adds $100 Million for Physical Education in Schools," *WYNC*, April 26, 2016, https://www.wnyc.org/story/mayors-budget-adds-100-million-physical-education-schools/.

4   "PE Works Year 4 Report 2018–2019," New York City Department of Education, https://infohub.nyced.org/reports/academics/annual-pe-works-reports/pe-works-year-4-report.

5   "Chancellor Carranza Announces $24 Million Investment in Health Ed Works," New York City Department of Education, https://www.schools.nyc.gov/about-us/news/announcements/contentdetails/2018/05/22/chancellor-carranza-announces-$24-million-investment-in-health-ed-works.

6   "Health Ed Works Year 1 Report 2019–2020," New York City Department of Education, https://infohub.nyced.org/reports/academics/health-ed-works/health-ed-works-year-1-report.

Chapter 3

1   Robert Beaglehole, et al., "Priority Actions for the Non-communicable Disease Crisis," *Lancet* 377, no. 9775 (April 23–27, 2011): 1438–1447, https://www.sciencedirect.com/science/article/pii/S0140673611603930.

2   Nikolaos Scarmeas, et al., "Physical Activity, Diet, and Risk of Alzheimer Disease," *Journal of the American Medical Association* 302, no. 6 (2009): 627–637, https://jamanetwork.com/journals/jama/fullarticle/184383.

3   "Shape Your Family's Habits," National Institutes of Health, https://newsinhealth.nih.gov/2013/02/shape-your-familys-habits.

4   "Promoting Health for Children and Adolescents," Centers for Disease Control, https://www.cdc.gov/chronicdisease/resources/publications/factsheets/children-health.htm.

5 Darren Warburton, et al., "Health Benefits of Physical Activity: The Evidence," *CMAJ* 174, no. 6 (March 14, 2006): 801–809, https://doi.org/10.1503/cmaj.051351.

6 David Lubans, et al. "Physical Activity for Cognitive and Mental Health in Youth: A Systematic Review of Mechanisms," *Pediatrics* 138, no. 3 (September 2016), https://doi.org/10.1542/peds.2016-1642.

7 "Childhood Nutrition Facts," Centers for Disease Control, https://www.cdc.gov/healthyschools/nutrition/facts.htm.

8 "Eating to Boost Energy," Harvard Medical School, https://www.health.harvard.edu/healthbeat/eating-to-boost-energy.

9 Rui Hai Liu, "Health benefits of fruit and vegetables are from additive and synergistic combinations of phytochemicals," *The American Journal of Clinical Nutrition* 78, no. 3 (September 2003): 517S–520S, https://doi.org/10.1093/ajcn/78.3.517S.

10 James Lee, et al., "Cigarette Smoking and Inflammation: Cellular and Molecular Mechanisms," *Journal of Dental Research* 91, no. 2 (February 1, 2012): 142–149, https://doi.org/10.1177/0022034511421200.

11 Andrew Parrott, et al., "Explaining the stress-inducing effects of nicotine to cigarette smokers," *Human Psychopharmacology*, March 5, 2012, https://doi.org/10.1002/hup.1247.

12 Andreas Jaehne, et al., "Effects of nicotine on sleep during consumption, withdrawal and replacement therapy," *Sleep Medicine Reviews* 13, no. 5 (October 2009): 363–377, https://doi.org/10.1016/j.smrv.2008.12.003.

13 Hui Chen, et al., "Cigarette Smoking and Brain Regulation of Energy Homeostasis," *Frontiers in Pharmacology 3, no. 147 (*2012), https://doi.org/10.3389/fphar.2012.00147.

14 Duncan P. Van Dusen, et al., "Associations of Physical Fitness and Academic Performance Among Schoolchildren," *Journal of School Health* 81, no. 12 (December 2011): 733–740, https://onlinelibrary.wiley.com/doi/abs/10.1111/j.1746-1561.2011.00652.x.

15 Ibid.

16 Centers for Disease Control, *Health and Academic Achievement* (Atlanta: U.S. Department of Health & Human Services, 2014), https://www.cdc.gov/healthyyouth/health_and_academics/pdf/health-academic-achievement.pdf.

17 Meg Walkley, et al., "Building Trauma-Informed Schools and Communities," *Children & Schools* 35, no. 2 (April 2013): 123–126, https://doi.org/10.1093/cs/cdt007.

18 François Trudeau, et al., "Physical Education, School Physical Activity, School Sports, and Academic Performance," *International Journal of Behavioral Nutrition and Physical Activity* 5, no. 10 (2008), https://ijbnpa.biomedcentral.com/articles/10.1186/1479-5868-5-10.

19 The Association of Supervision and Curriculum Development, *The Learning Compact Redefined: A Call to Action* (2007), http://www.ascd.org/learningcompact.

Case Study: Principal in Action—Solomon P. Ortiz Elementary School, Brownsville, Texas

1 Susan A. Everson, et al., "Epidemiologic Evidence for the Relation Between Socioeconomic Status and Depression, Obesity, and Diabetes," Journal of Psychosomatic Research 53, no. 4 (2002): 891–895, https://doi.org/10.1016/S0022-3999(02)00303-3.

2 Dan Solomon, "The FBI's List of the Most Dangerous Cities in Texas," *Texas Monthly*, January 22, 2015, https://www.texasmonthly.com/the-daily-post/the-fbis-list-of-the-most-dangerous-cities-in-texas/.

3 "2019 Accountability Rating System," Texas Education Agency, https://tea.texas.gov/Student_Testing_and_Accountability/Accountability/State_Accountability/Performance_Reporting/2019_Accountability_Rating_System.

4 Ibid.

5 "Reward School Case Studies," Texas Education Agency, https://tea.texas.gov/Student_Testing_and_Accountability/Monitoring_and_Interventions/School_Improvement_and_Support/Reward_School_Case_Studies.

6 "America's Best Urban Schools Award Winners," National Center for Urban School Transformation, https://ncust.com/previous-americas-best-urban-schools-award-winners/.

Chapter 4

1 Steven H. Woolf, et al., "Life Expectancy and Mortality Rates in the United States, 1959–2017," *Journal of the American Medical Association* 322, no. 20 (2019): 1996–2016, https://doi.org/10.1001/jama.2019.16932.

2   Institute of Medicine, *The Healthcare Imperative: Lowering Costs and Improving Outcomes* (Washington, DC: National Academies Press, 2010), https://www.ncbi.nlm.nih.gov/books/NBK53914/.

3   Centers for Medicare & Medicaid Services, *National Health Expenditures Highlights* (2016), https://www.cms.gov/Research-Statistics-Data-and-Systems/Statistics-Trends-and-Reports/NationalHealthExpendData/downloads/highlights.pdf.

4   George Miller, et al., "Quantifying National Spending on Wellness and Prevention," *Advances in Health Economics and Health Services Research* 19 (2008): 1–24, https://pubmed.ncbi.nlm.nih.gov/19548511/.

Chapter 5

1   Albert Bandura, "Health Promotion from the Perspective of Social Cognitive Theory," *Psychology & Health* 13, no. 4 (1998): 623–649, https://www.tandfonline.com/doi/abs/10.1080/08870449808407422.

2   "What is SEL?", CASEL, https://casel.org/what-is-sel/.

3   Mary Ann Pentz, "Effective Prevention Programs for Tobacco Use," *Nicotine & Tobacco Research* 1, no. 1 Supplement (1999): S99–S107, https://academic.oup.com/ntr/article-abstract/1/Suppl_1/S99/1086492.

4   David Schultz, et al., "Effects of the Flipped Classroom Model on Student Performance for Advanced Placement High School Chemistry Students," *Journal of Chemical Education* 91, no. 9 (July 2014): 1334–1339, https://doi.org/10.1021/ed400868x.

5   "National Health Education Standards," Centers for Disease Control, https://www.cdc.gov/healthyschools/sher/standards/index.htm.

6   "Characteristics of an Effective Health Education Curriculum," Centers for Disease Control, https://www.cdc.gov/healthyschools/sher/characteristics/index.htm.

7   Centers for Disease Control, *Results from the School Health Policies and Practices Study 2014* (2015). Table 1.15 average across 8 health education topics, https://www.cdc.gov/healthyyouth/data/shpps/pdf/shpps-508-final_101315.pdf.

8   Washington State Health Care Authority (Developed by Joe Neigel, Monroe Community Coalition Coordinator), *Prevention Tools: What Works, What Doesn't* (2016), https://www.theathenaforum.org/best-practices-toolkit-prevention-tools-what-works-what-doesnt.

9   Melanie B. Tannenbaum, et al., "Appealing to Fear: A Meta-analysis of
    Fear Appeal Effectiveness and Theories," *Psychological Bulletin* 141, no. 6
    (2015): 1178–1204, https://psycnet.apa.org/record/2015-48611-002.

10 Noel T. Brewer, et al., "Pictorial Cigarette Warnings Increase Quitting:
    a Comment on Kok et al.," *Health Psychology Review* 12, no. 2 (2018):
    129–132, https://www.tandfonline.com/doi/abs/10.1080/17437199.2018.
    1445544.

Chapter 6

1   Centers for Disease Control, *Results from the School Health Policies and
    Practices Study 2014* (2015) Tables 1.3, 2.9, 2.15, 1.10, 1.11, 2.14, 1.12, 2.27,
    2.33, 3.14, https://www.cdc.gov/healthyyouth/data/shpps/pdf/shpps-
    508-final_101315.pdf.

2   "Shape Your Family's Habits," National Institutes of Health, https://
    newsinhealth.nih.gov/2013/02/shape-your-familys-habits.

3   "Promoting Health for Children and Adolescents," Centers for Disease
    Control, https://www.cdc.gov/chronicdisease/resources/publications/
    factsheets/children-health.htm.

4   Centers for Disease Control, *Results from the School Health Policies and
    Practices Study 2014* (2015) Tables 1.3, 2.9, 2.15, 1.10, 1.11, 2.14, 1.12, 2.27,
    2.33, 3.14, https://www.cdc.gov/healthyyouth/data/shpps/pdf/shpps-
    508-final_101315.pdf.

5   Centers for Disease Control, *Results from the School Health Policies and
    Practices Study 2014* (2015) Tables 1.3, 2.9, 2.15, 1.10, 1.11, 2.14, 1.12, 2.27,
    2.33, 3.14, https://www.cdc.gov/healthyyouth/data/shpps/pdf/shpps-
    508-final_101315.pdf.

6   SHAPE America—Society of Health and Physical Educators, *Using
    Physical Activity as Punishment and/or Behavior Management* (2009),
    https://www.shapeamerica.org/uploads/pdfs/positionstatements/
    using-physical-activity-as-punishment-2009.pdf.

7   Ibid.

Case Study: District in Action—Goose Creek CISD, Baytown, Texas

1   "CATCH Promise Spotlight: Goose Creek CISD," CATCH Global
    Foundation, https://catchinfo.org/spotlight/goose-creek-cisd/.

Chapter 7

1   "Youth Tobacco Use: Results From the National Youth Tobacco Survey (2019)," U.S. Food and Drug Administration and Centers for Disease Control, https://www.fda.gov/tobacco-products/youth-and-tobacco/youth-tobacco-use-results-national-youth-tobacco-survey. Prior years available at: https://www.cdc.gov/tobacco/data_statistics/surveys/nyts/index.htm.

2   "Youth and Tobacco Use (2019)," Centers for Disease Control, https://www.cdc.gov/tobacco/data_statistics/fact_sheets/youth_data/tobacco_use/index.htm.

3   Office of the Surgeon General. *E-cigarette Use among Youth and Young Adults: A Report of the Surgeon General* (Washington, DC: U.S. Department of Health and Human Services, Centers for Disease Control and Prevention, 2016), https://www.cdc.gov/tobacco/data_statistics/sgr/e-cigarettes/pdfs/2016_sgr_entire_report_508.pdf.

4   Brian A. Primack et al., "Initiation of Traditional Cigarette Smoking after Electronic Cigarette Use among Tobacco-Naïve U.S. Young Adults," *The American Journal of Medicine* 131, no. 4 (2017): 443.e1 - 443.e92017, https://doi.org/10.1016/j.amjmed.2017.11.005.

5   Office of the Surgeon General. *E-cigarette Use among Youth and Young Adults: A Report of the Surgeon General* (Washington, DC: U.S. Department of Health and Human Services, Centers for Disease Control and Prevention, 2016), https://www.cdc.gov/tobacco/data_statistics/sgr/e-cigarettes/pdfs/2016_sgr_entire_report_508.pdf.

6   Eric R. Kandel et al., "A Molecular Basis for Nicotine as a Gateway Drug," *New England Journal of Medicine* 371, no. 10 (September 4, 2014): 932–943, https://doi.org/10.1056/NEJMsa1405092.

7   Sally H. Adams et al., "Medical Vulnerability of Young Adults to Severe COVID-19 Illness—Data From the National Health Interview Survey," *Journal of Adolescent Health* (published online July 13, 2020), https://doi.org/10.1016/j.jadohealth.2020.06.025.

8   Roengrudee Patanavanich et al., "Smoking Is Associated With COVID-19 Progression: A Meta-analysis," *Nicotine & Tobacco Research* (published online May 11, 2020), https://www.ncbi.nlm.nih.gov/pmc/articles/PMC7239135/.

9   "Outbreak of Lung Injury Associated with the Use of E-cigarette, or Vaping, Products (February 25, 2020)," Centers for Disease Control, https://www.cdc.gov/tobacco/basic_information/e-cigarettes/severe-lung-disease.html.

10 Tony Plohetski, "Austin Student Killed Over Vaping Drugs, Sources Say," *Statesman*, March 27, 2019, https://www.statesman.com/news/20190327/austin-student-killed-over-vaping-drugs-sources-say.

11 Robert K. Jackler et al., "JUUL Advertising Over its First Three Years on the Market," *Stanford Research into the Impact of Tobacco Advertising* (January 31, 2019), http://tobacco.stanford.edu/tobacco_main/publications/JUUL_Marketing_Stanford.pdf.

12 Jeffrey G. Willett et al., "Recognition, Use and Perceptions of JUUL Among Youth and Young Adults," *Tobacco Control* 28, no. 1 (2018), https://tobaccocontrol.bmj.com/content/28/1/115.

13 "The Flavor Trap," Campaign for Tobacco-Free Kids, https://www.tobaccofreekids.org/microsites/flavortrap/#findings.

14 "PUFF Krush Add-On Pre-Filled Vape Pods 24 pk," Indigo Distribution, https://indigodistro.com/puff-krush-add-on-pre-filled-vape-pods/.

15 Lloyd D. Johnston et al., *Monitoring the Future National Survey on Drug Use 1975–2018* (Ann Arbor: Institute for Social Research, University of Michigan, 2019), http://www.monitoringthefuture.org/pubs/monographs/mtf-overview2018.pdf.

16 CATCH Global Foundation, CATCH My Breath Youth E-Cigarette Prevention, 2018–19 Evaluation Report (2019).

17 "Quick Facts on the Risks of E-cigarettes for Kids, Teens, and Young Adults (2019)," Centers for Disease Control, https://www.cdc.gov/tobacco/basic_information/e-cigarettes/Quick-Facts-on-the-Risks-of-E-cigarettes-for-Kids-Teens-and-Young-Adults.html.

18 "'Covered' Tobacco Products and Roll-Your-Own/Cigarette Tobacco Labeling and Warning Statement Requirements (2019)," U.S. Food and Drug Administration, https://www.fda.gov/TobaccoProducts/Labeling/Labeling/ucm524470.htm.

19 "Testimony: Examining the Response to Lung Illnesses and Rising Youth Electronic Cigarette Use (November 13, 2019)," U.S. Food and Drug Administration, https://www.fda.gov/news-events/congressional-testimony/examining-response-lung-illnesses-and-rising-youth-electronic-cigarette-use-11132019.

20 World Health Organization, *WHO Report on the Global Tobacco Epidemic*, 2008 (Geneva: World Health Organization, 2008), https://www.who.int/tobacco/mpower/mpower_report_full_2008.pdf.

21 Aviva Shen, "The Disastrous Legacy of Nancy Reagan's 'Just Say
    No' Campaign," *ThinkProgress*, March 6, 2016, https://thinkprogress.
    org/the-disastrous-legacy-of-nancy-reagans-just-say-no-campaign-
    fd24570bf109/.

Chapter 8

1   Jane Meredith Adams, "Lawsuit Agreement to Force Schools to Provide
    Physical Education," *EdSource*, February 1, 2015, https://edsource.
    org/2015/lawsuit-agreement-to-force-schools-to-provide-physical-
    education/73544.

2   U.S. Department of Health and Human Services, *2008 Physical Activity
    Guidelines for Americans* (2008), https://health.gov/paguidelines/pdf/
    paguide.pdf.

3   "2011 Compendium of Physical Activities: A Second Update
    of Codes and MET Values," *Medicine and Science in Sports and
    Exercise* 43, no. 8 (2011): 1575–1581, https://sites.google.com/site/
    compendiumofphysicalactivities/.

4   Ibid.

5   Centers for Disease Control, *Results from the School Health Policies
    and Practices Study 2014* (2015), Table 2.8, https://www.cdc.gov/
    healthyyouth/data/shpps/pdf/shpps-508-final_101315.pdf.

6   Centers for Disease Control, *Strategies to Improve the Quality of
    Physical Education* (2010), https://www.cdc.gov/healthyschools/pecat/
    quality_pe.pdf.

7   CATCH Global Foundation internal data.

8   "This Is Your Brain on Exercise: Why Physical Exercise (Not Mental
    Games) Might Be the Best Way to Keep Your Mind Sharp," Open
    Culture, http://www.openculture.com/2018/03/brain-on-exercise.html.

9   Centers for Disease Control, *Results from the School Health Policies
    and Practices Study 2014* (2015), Table 2.8, https://www.cdc.gov/
    healthyyouth/data/shpps/pdf/shpps-508-final_101315.pdf.

10 Ibid.

11 CATCH Global Foundation internal data.

12 CATCH Global Foundation internal data.

Chapter 9

1   Dara R. Musher-Eizenman, et al., "Emerald Dragon Bites vs Veggie Beans: Fun Food Names Increase Children's Consumption of Novel Healthy Foods," *Journal of Early Childhood Research* 9, no. 3 (2011): 191–195, https://doi.org/10.1177/1476718X10366729.

2   Centers for Disease Control, *Results from the School Health Policies and Practices Study 2014* (2015), Tables 3.7, 3.10, 3.8, 3.9, https://www.cdc.gov/healthyyouth/data/shpps/pdf/shpps-508-final_101315.pdf.

3   Centers for Disease Control, *Results from the School Health Policies and Practices Study 2014* (2015), Tables 3.7, 3.10, 3.8, 3.9, https://www.cdc.gov/healthyyouth/data/shpps/pdf/shpps-508-final_101315.pdf.

Chapter 10

1   "CATCH Research: Understanding the Importance of Health Education in Schools," CATCH Global Foundation, https://catchinfo.org/research/.

2   Rodrigo S. Reis, et al., "Scaling Up Physical Activity Interventions Worldwide: Stepping Up to Larger and Smarter Interventions to Get People Moving," *The Lancet* 388, no. 10051 (September 24–30 2016): 1337–1348, https://www.sciencedirect.com/journal/the-lancet/vol/388/issue/10051.

3   Steven H. Kelder et al., "A Middle School Program to Prevent E-Cigarette Use: A Pilot Study of "CATCH My Breath," *Public Health Reports* 135, 2 (January 2020): 220–229, https://doi.org/10.1177/0033354919900887.

4   CATCH Global Foundation internal data.

Chapter 11

1   "Schools and Staffing Survey," National Center for Education Statistics (weekly hour totals multiplied by 36 weeks in average school year), https://nces.ed.gov/surveys/sass/tables/sass0708_005_t1n.asp.

2   Centers for Disease Control, *Results from the School Health Policies and Practices Study 2014* (2015), Table 1.13 (for elementary schools, multiplied average hours for each topic by percentage of schools requiring that topic and assume two doses of each topic in six-year K–5 sequence), https://www.cdc.gov/healthyyouth/data/shpps/pdf/shpps-508-final_101315.pdf.

Made in the USA
Coppell, TX
25 July 2021

59472364R00134